THIN
IS A
STATE OF MIND

Nancy Bryan, Ph.D.

THIN
IS A
STATE OF MIND

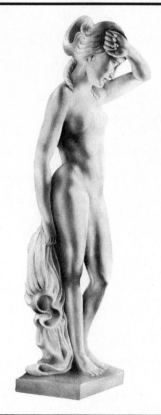

CompCare®
publications

Minneapolis, Minnesota
Newport Beach, California

Bryan, Nancy L.
   Thin is a state of mind.

   Bibliography: p.
   1. Reducing — Psychological aspects.
2. Mind and body.
I. Title.
RM222.2.B8 1982   613.2'5'019   81-22168
ISBN 0-89638-055-6   AACR2
ISBN 0-89638-056-4 (pbk.)

   Inquiries, orders, and catalog requests should be addressed to
   CompCare Publications
   2415 Annapolis Lane
   Minneapolis, Minnesota 55441
   Call toll free 800/328-3330.
   (Minnesota residents 612/559-4800.)

For Fred

and Janet
    Bonnie
    Sara
    Katy
    Liz
    Heather
    Sean
    Ulysses

Contents

Preface

This may be the first book on weight loss that honestly considers its readers to be intelligent people. It was written for you if you are tired of the nonsense I call the fairy-tale approach to dieting. If you understand that losing weight is a physiological event, not a wish upon a star, and are ready to get on with whatever realistically needs to be done to be rid of the problem once and for all, this book can and will help you.

I'm sure you have seen and read enough to be disillusioned with the dead-end "try-harder" philosophy of most diet books. This isn't a diet book. It is better than that, for it will tell you what you need to know to be successful with whatever diet plan you have ever (fruitlessly) tried to follow. Other books tell you what to *do*; this book assumes that if you could follow those instructions, you would *already* be thin and have little need for a book telling you how to get that way.

The point is that right now you *aren't* able to follow the directions. For a variety of very good reasons, many internal obstacles are keeping you from your goal. This book will discuss these subliminal obstacles (that is, the constant directions you give yourself to stay fat) in great detail and show that, once they are gone, any excess weight will come off almost without your trying—certainly without any of the standard agonies we have come to expect from "being on a diet."

This book is an authentic self-help manual, written to give others as much help as writing it is giving me. It provides the one quality in short supply among today's diet books—wisdom—though it aims to be nothing more than an honest account of the stepping stones as well as the blind alleys on the path of gradual self-discovery. (Sources of quotations are cited in a list of references at the back of the book.)

I was one of those ambitious young women who simply couldn't comprehend why the same direct, informed, *capable* attack that brought me success in other areas of my life should fail so utterly when applied to overweight. Maybe you are a similar person. We have all been exposed to an encyclopedic range of information (the outer instructions, as it were) for solving the problem of overweight. But since, even with all this knowledge, millions of people *still* are fatter than they want to be, something must be very wrong with our approach to the problem.

This book formulates what I call the inner instructions, those principles which, when understood, will make the outer instructions much easier—in fact, almost trivial—to follow. This book is written to help people who think their only problem is to weigh what they want to weigh, when the real question—unknown to them, perhaps—is how to bring into being the life they want and the person they want living in it.

Acknowledgments

This book's existence is owed to the many kinds of help and encouragement I have been given by many people. I take great pleasure in expressing my thanks to at least some of those people here.

To Eric Mader, my first "patient," whose 70-pound weight loss startled us both and convinced me that the validity of these ideas was not merely a figment of my imagination.

To Susan Newton, Ph.D., founder of Marina Hypnosciences of Los Angeles, for whose remarkable insights my gratitude and indebtedness are beyond measure; and to Alexandra Beckett, who continued Susan's work with wit and acuity.

To Thich An Thanh, M.D., for his gentle insistence and rigorous compassion while he taught me how to make my body fully healthy.

To Fred Dorsett, who unfailingly knew when to give an encouraging pat on the back and when an encouraging kick in the pants.

To Daisy Lindner, R.N., who selflessly cheered and encouraged me—to the limits of all human patience—during a difficult time.

To Steven Polin, M.D., and Robert Fenichel, M.D., for medical advice generously given.

To my dear friend Becky Goodman, whom I have always considered my own personal Fairy Godmother, for hours of shared laughter.

To Cathy Edgerly, formerly my exercise teacher and still my friend, with whom I have spent many pleasurable hours exchanging ideas and trying out my fledgling thoughts on the body/mind relationship.

To Rose Kattlove, a highly sympathetic (and virtually indefatigable) listener in fat times and thin.

To Jane Browne, my wise and wonderful agent, for listening to an idea and transforming it into a reality.

To Bill Alexander, for believing in the book in the first place and for cheering me on during the writing of it.

To Diana Mann, whose own warmth transformed the mere business transaction of typing the manuscript into a rewarding and nourishing personal relationship.

One acknowledgment of indebtedness that it grieves me not to be able to make in person is that to my late college writing teacher, Frederick L. Mulhauser, whose vision of quality in written expression and whose extraordinary integrity have served as personal lodestars throughout my adult life.

This book's virtues are owed to the high quality of help I have received from many knowledgeable, compassionate sources, both those mentioned and many others as well. The book's defects, I hasten to admit, are mine alone.

THE PROBLEM

1
The Wrong Way to Solve Problems

Whole sight; or all the rest is desolation.
John Fowles, *Daniel Martin*

My credentials for writing this book are impeccable. I have been obsessed with the subject of overweight all my life, and this book is as inevitable a result of my concern as if I were a professional tennis player writing about having spent my entire life on the courts. Naturally, I have always been an avid student of diet books. Being fat and wanting desperately to be thin was what I worried over every day of my waking life. I became an adult, went to school for many years, earned a Ph.D., was married, had children, held jobs, and so forth—but no matter what I was doing, two alternating thoughts turned repeatedly inside my head: "I'm fat and I want to be thin," and "I'm hungry and I want to eat."

Of course I and the millions of Americans like me want to be thin; we would be happier and healthier that way. But as it stands now we're made to feel guilty about being fat (the actual poundage is irrelevant) and have become convinced that it is somehow our fault. In our culture there is no other readily available way to think. Two things most people in America agree on are (1) fat is ugly, and (2) people who are fat are to blame for being that way. As Dr. Jean Mayer of Harvard University said, "Obesity, almost alone among all the pathologic conditions [including alcoholism and drug addiction], remains a moral issue."

The American diet industry is definitely Big Business; catering to the nation's estimated 60 or 70 million overweight people (in other words, between 30 and 40 percent of the population) has become a $10 billion concern. But it is a melancholy giant, with more than a passing resemblance to the Why-Johnny-Can't-Read and Why-Is-My-Sex-Life-So-Lousy industries, which attempt to capitalize on paralyzing human worries and harass them to death with anxious Solutions and Techniques. We don't like to acknowledge that some problems might become more manageable, might even resolve themselves, if they were treated with a little benign neglect. In other words, it is our zeal to overwhelm problems with solutions (more and more technical and mechanical) that *guarantees* the problems will never, ever disappear. Nationwide statistics indicate that only about 2 percent of obese people ever reach normal weight and maintain it over an extended period of time. The relentless merchandising of guilt feelings concerning a persistent human condition is such that overweight people have virtually become the victims of the American diet industry rather than its beneficiaries.

Yes, we need all the detailed information we can get on how things really work. The good news is that, for perhaps the first time in history, enough of the factual, technical parts of the puzzle seem to be in place. But the facts themselves aren't enough. If the huge bulk of factual diet literature were in itself sufficient to make the problem disappear, it would *already* have gone away.

I am sometimes greatly distressed to find myself a writer of what may seem to be a "diet book"; one editor remarked on the difficulties of any book's survival on "this crowded and glutted track." I would probably be unable to muster the courage to add my contribution at all if it were not for three convictions:

1. There is a coherence, even elegance, to the entire problem of obesity that can be reassuring and encouraging to an overweight person struggling toward a personal solution to the problem.

2. Nearly all the books written so far exhibit similar cultural blind spots that degrade the usefulness of their advice.

3. No book has yet been written that truly sees the whole. The greatest single value of this book is that it does.

The immense value of being able to see the orderliness of the whole is that seeing the whole is the first step toward accepting the universe, and accepting the universe is the first step toward solving the problem. Overweight people often suffer from a pervasive sense of hopelessness, the result of a deeply held suspicion that the universe does not make sense. (If the universe were rational, surely one would not be required to be fat.) In fact, the notion that there *is* a coherent whole is probably astonishing to those who view their lifelong weight problem as nothing more than one disastrous, unexpected event after another. Anyone who has ever dieted strenuously, only to have the lost weight reassert itself a while later, questions not only his brand of cottage cheese but the overall justice of the world as well. When the solution to a pressing problem continues to elude you, you will be either (at best) thoroughly discouraged or (at worst) demoralized enough to give up altogether.

The problem of obesity in our society is a very complex issue. It is like trying to open a combination lock. If you're an earnest dieter, you've probably already done the equivalent of turning one or two tumblers, but the lock still hasn't opened. That doesn't mean you've failed; it means only that you haven't discovered the missing numbers. This book will identify them for you and help you understand what's gone wrong in your previous attempts to make the problem disappear.

Books on losing weight can be divided into two types: those addressed to the body alone (the "hardware" approach) and those addressed to the mind (the "software" approach). The first type climb to the top of the best-seller lists with regularity because the diets they prescribe seem to work—*as long as you stay on them.* As soon as you quit, the weight comes right back. The second type are never as popular because their advice seems more diffuse, something hard to translate into pounds lost in a week's time. Both are, sooner or later, blind alleys for the large majority of their readers.

This situation is very much like two gangs of laborers trying to dig a tunnel from opposite sides of a mountain. Both teams break their backs moving dirt, but the tunnel—the goal they are both working toward—does not and cannot exist until they meet. Books on the body alone will never solve the problem, nor will books on the mind alone. We can see the whole only by grasping the notion of the *bodymind*—the body that is a visible manifestation, an inevitable result, of a group of interacting subliminally held ideas. The current status of our overall understanding of obesity is the equivalent of the last cubic yards of earth preventing the two groups of diggers from joining their efforts in the achievement of the tunnel. We should now be more than ready to remove that obstacle and shine the light of a new discipline on the intricacies of the problem.

This book is written from the perspective of cybernetics, the study of goal-seeking mechanisms. For our purposes the term *goal seeking* can be thought of as exactly equivalent to *problem solving.* By virtue of your very being, you are naturally a goal-seeking or problem-solving mechanism. The only meaningful questions are, What do you need to know to release your own inborn problem-solving abilities? and What obstacles do you have to recognize and remove in order to be successful?

E. W. Dijkstra, a cybernetics theoretician, once commented in an interview on the necessity of the proper mental tools for the efficient solution of any problem:

It's very illuminating to think about the fact that some—at most four hundred years ago—professors at European universities would tell the brilliant students that if they were very diligent, it was not impossible to learn how to do long division. . . . You see, the poor guys had to do it in Roman numerals. Now here you see in a nutshell what a difference there is in good and bad notation . . . because tools have such a profound influence on the thinking habits of the people who are trying to use them.

As we work on the problem of obesity, we continue to sidetrack ourselves in two ways: first, we use the information we have inappropriately; second, we choose inappropriate problem-solving methods. We do not yet comprehend that the facts we know are not the deepest things there are to be known. We foolishly tend to see given phenomena as ends in themselves rather than as concrete illustrations of underlying principles, as if we thought light bulbs generated light. In dieting this becomes an insistence on certain foods, certain types or amounts of exercise, certain ways of behaving, and so forth. If we believe that grapefruit has special properties, or that we must eat only three times a day and only while seated in our dining room, we have surely missed the point. We need to lose our intentness on the facts themselves and develop a keen curiosity about the deeper truths or principles, the organic connections between facts that link them into a single orderly whole.

When you don't understand the fundamental principles illustrated by the particular diet book you are reading at the moment, you are forced into great (and unnecessary) literalmindedness about following the method, which feels much like walking along a very narrow footpath in the dark. Following the directions to the letter is the only thing that seems safe to do. The same is true of writers of diet books, unfortunately; without understanding the general principles which their particular methods merely illustrate, they are forced into an irritating and gratuitous dogmatism: do it my way or you'll be sorry. Because this book is about general principles, I hope it can help you understand and be successful with whatever favorite diet method you may have used but couldn't make work permanently.

To solve a problem of any kind, the first thing needed is to find out if there is a hierarchy to the parts of the problem—in other words, if there are certain things you can't solve until you've solved other things. Without that crucial information you could waste a lot of time in blind alleys. Oddly enough, very, very few of the thousands of works on obesity have ever tried to discover an order to the parts of the problem. However, there is one: (1) unworkable view of reality; (2) anxiety; (3) faulty body chemistry; (4) bad habits. Since each of these in turn works to bring about the next, it is impossible to work productively on the second part of the problem without having solved the first, on the third without having solved both the first and second, and so on.

It is important that we develop an appreciation of how to solve problems by indirection. One of our cultural blind spots is that we are too much in love with "trying." We seem to believe that no achievement could possibly be worthwhile unless it required valiant effort. But Timothy Gallwey defined the Inner Game as an enterprise in which there are no "have-to's." A *New Times* article about Gallwey neatly summarized his attractive, sensible philosophy: "He says that one of the greatest deterrents to doing anything well is trying to do it well. 'Nobody ever tries to turn a light on,' Gallwey explained. . . . 'You only try when there is some assumption of doubt. [The Zen term *effortless effort*] just refers to the economic use of one's energy.' "

Our normal American method for solving problems just doesn't work with personal issues such as overweight. All the effort we think is needed for "controlling" the rampant desires of overweight people shows merely that we do not understand anything about how to achieve that peaceful inner state that makes this kind of outer control unnecessary. Most diet books speak only to the self as it *might be* (if you *could* follow the instructions, if you *were* able to control yourself). None of them attempts to meet you where you are. None of them tries to bridge that enormous gap between the resistant, angry, frustrated person who is still fat and the exhilarated, joyful one who isn't. They invariably ignore the shadow self—defiant, blind, and needy—that controls compulsive behavior. In fact, the writers of cheery diet books do not seem to understand the streak of defiance their words call up in the minds of overweight readers. Whenever I read a book or article that ended with the admonition, "Be sure to see your doctor before following this or any other diet plan," I always mentally replied, "The hell I will." This hidden defiance is not unique to me; it is a nearly universal quality among overweight people. The reason for it is not at all difficult to discover. All overweight people either *need* to or very much *want* to eat more food than is good for them—an activity which their culture considers shameful. The fact that a person will be censured for his or her wants never makes those wants go away but only makes the person defensive about them and openly or secretly resentful of the criticism. Upbraiding a fat person for overeating is probably the most effective way of making sure that he or she will need to keep on doing it.

We hear a lot about motivation, as if it's something one should do or a quality one should possess. Whenever a doctor lectured me about motivation, I shuddered inside, convinced that however much of it I had, it was not going to be enough to keep me on my diet during moments of temptation. (I was right, of course, but only because I chose to listen to, believe, and therefore make true that frightened, self-belittling view.) In reality, motivation consists almost entirely of the working out in time of a goal that is unimpeded by neurotic personal obstacles. Motivation is a by-product of becoming engrossed in something else, and gradually becoming able to dispel your anxiety about your weight. We all talk about willpower at great length, wishing we had more of it than we do. But we can only exercise self-discipline—the outward manifestation of inner control—as long as our hearts and minds are in accord. When we can't control our behavior, it means only that our desires and our will are not working together. We can learn to make them work together, and when they do, the "problem" vanishes for all practical purposes. We have been conditioned to believe that dieting is unpleasant, whereas it is really just another human process. It is a time of learning, beginning to see what you do to cause your overweight, getting to know your body, and teaching your mind the facts you need to understand your body better.

If you accept yourself as a learning mechanism, you can relax and let the learning happen to you—if you are lucky enough not to share the widespread cultural bias about failure. An essential component of all cybernetic systems is *feedback,* which is defined as information about past behavior given to the system to help improve its present performance. In other words, the essence of a cybernetic system is to gradually improve itself by means of an increasingly educated process of trial and error. In our culture we dislike the notion of trial and error as a learning device because we can't abide the "error" part: we think it's shameful and unacceptable to fail. But this is just another cultural blind spot. J. A. Winter's book *Why We Get Sick: The Origins of Illness and Anxiety* contains a chapter entitled "The Importance of Making Mistakes," with a subheading called "The Mistake as a Basic Learning Pattern," in which he explains that "one makes a mistake; by correcting the mistake, one gets closer to the goal; the process is repeated as long as necessary." Or, as Baba Ram Dass once remarked in an interview, "The whole spiritual journey is a continuous falling on your face."

For my own part I now understand that the worst "failures" of my life were the richest learning experiences, and the episodes of utter humiliation did more to get me on the track toward eventual success than anything else could possibly have done. It is crucial that we come to understand that errors are opportunities to learn and improve (in fact, the pointers along the path toward success). Failing too often, with demoralizing effects, is not *wrong;* it means simply that one's aim was slightly too high at the beginning.

Lack of detail is the most common and most debilitating flaw among diet writings. Very few are sufficiently meticulous in their descriptions of successful weight loss so that a reader starting from square one could learn step by step what needs to be done. They also misrepresent the process in another fundamental way. When people who have lost weight themselves get around to writing diet books, they are fooled into believing that what they *did* (how many calories, how much exercise) was what counted, not who they were and how they got there.

Anyone's successful, long-term weight loss involves only one event of any importance: a change, at a deep level, of how the world is perceived. Eric Berne has observed that there is a certain point in the recovery of every neurotic patient marked by a change in perception. Before it the person feels himself to be sick, and after it he is aware that he is getting well. Berne claimed that no lasting progress was possible until the patient had reached the latter state. When this event occurs for a fat person, it produces what I call the thin mind-set. After the person has the thin mind-set, his subconscious mind simply goes about following his own deeply programmed instructions to become thin.

Though our culture believes in "doing," it is really "being" that matters; the idea is prior to its execution in reality. When I became thin, only in a very limited sense was my diet the agent of change. A more fundamental, primary cause was that I became a person to whom the excess weight simply didn't belong. An overweight person is obese not only in terms of poundage; his or her whole being (relationships, inner feelings, self-image) has become short-circuited through food. Because we are goal-seeking mechanisms, we need to have the goal clearly in mind before we can begin to pursue it effectively. The clarity of our idea depends critically on the quality of clarity in our minds—clarity we achieve in proportion to how well we align ourselves with the universe in a spirit of serenity.

We all need support from within. If we are overweight, we need to construct for ourselves personalities more able to cope with the temptations of food. We can best do this by developing a meditative habit of mind, which could be thought of as a way to feed our insides so we are more able to cope with not feeding our outsides. We probably cannot hear advice until it is phrased in such a way, tuned to such a wavelength, that it enters our beings nearly unaware. We still await the authentic voice—the Walt Whitman of the overupholstered—that can celebrate what it feels like to be us and tell us what we can do, what we must endure, what we can cherish about ourselves. The authentic voice will come from within. This book will tell you what to listen for, and how to listen well.

2
My Own Experience

If you want to write the truth, you must write about yourself. I am the only real truth I know.

Jean Rhys

This chapter is a specialized type of autobiography, neither a breathless my-binges-can-top-yours confessional nor a reformed-sinner moral tract (though at times it may seem to have elements of both). It is rather an account, as honest as I can possibly make it, of the experiences I lived through as a chronic dieter/binger/food-obsessed compulsive overeater, then my account of what I finally saw these experiences *meant*. My experiences might well have been called fragments in search of a pattern, for that is how they appeared to me at the time— chaotic fragments of what under less.exigent circumstances might have been a successful life. The chapter ends with how I learned to solve my problem, though my failures and flounderings are the more valuable and instructive parts of the story I have to tell.

As I said before, my credentials are impeccable. I am still unable to pass by one of those "I-lost-100-pounds-with-Ayds" ads without reading it through on the spot, and I have never glimpsed a height-weight table without spending a few moments finding out its opinion about how much a medium-frame five-foot-six female should weigh. When Dr. Rubin's questionnaire in *Forever Thin* asked what could be paraphrased as, "Do you tend to remember social events by what food was served?" I would once have answered, "Of course! What else is there to notice?" I am a sister under the skin to every overweight person I have ever met; I have never heard a "fat story" I couldn't identify with. I give you my story here not (God knows) because the world needs another tale of out-of-control eating and guilt, but because, first, in a basic sense it is all I have to give; and second, if I "tell it truly," as Ernest Hemingway liked to say, to the extent that I am willing to be honest, you will be able to identify with me—not only with my former problem but also with my having ultimately found a solution. I am convinced that all "fat people" or "formerly fat people" live life scripts of startling similarity. While the events of our lives may be different, the feelings these events elicit in us are remarkably alike.

To someone who is not an overeater my stated resolve to be thoroughly honest in telling my tale may not seem particularly remarkable or courageous. Actually, it isn't hard for me to be honest now, but at another stage in my life it would have been utterly impossible. My all-consuming desire to overeat was once the aspect of myself I would never have dreamed of revealing, though paradoxically it loomed larger in my secret life than anything else—a hidden, unacknowledged iceberg. As with many other fat people, my being too proud to admit and talk about my problem isolated me in self-consciousness, making me suffer all alone.

Like every other overeater I know, I never ate normally; I spent my entire life either dieting or binging. Never during my life did my behavior make sense to me. I knew that I didn't want to be fat, but being fat was controlled by how much one ate, and since I couldn't stop eating, what else was there to say? I did know that my eating made me ashamed of myself, which is why I hid candy wrappers and cookie boxes from my grade school years on. My fat self, the result of the eating, caused me further shame, which is why I was so humiliated by everything from "fatty fatty two-by-four" when I was eight to a snide salesgirl's sidelong glance in a department store fitting room when I was thirty.

My entire life was once organized around protective rituals: keeping my arms folded over my stomach for camouflage, never engaging in sports if an audience was present, refusing to buy myself clothes whenever I weighed more than a certain acceptable figure, eating irreproachably at family mealtimes, and so forth. Life was primarily a holding action, fending off criticism before it happened, assuaging hurts or disappointments with food afterward. In that sense my life was a continuing ad hoc performance, an improvisation to shore me up against disaster. I was told I had a good mind, and I used it to console myself for the deficiencies of my body, but it was never enough, never truly and finally satisfying.

In retrospect, I have begun to see the pattern, and I offer my experience to you so that you may discover yours. The reason I could never see what it all meant before was that I was examining all the wrong evidence, using all the wrong measuring tools. I had not yet been led to ask the right questions. The coherence and order of my life did not become clear to me until I was able to consider it as *inner* experience. When I saw it only as a miscellaneous collection of motley events that *happened to me* rather than as the feelings with which I habitually reacted, I was as absurdly limited in my tools for understanding as Hansel and Gretel searching for crumbs. In short, the markers I plan to show you are not the outward events of my life, which are distinctly secondary to the reactions to people and events that I chose to repeat again and again under entirely different outward circumstances. These reactions became "me," my personality, my chronic inner environment that made obesity consciousness an inevitable fact of my life. The other significant part of my history is biochemical: confusing, anomalous bodily facts which I once couldn't understand (my moodiness, my lack of energy, my getting sick on Dr. Atkins' diet) but which I see now to be part of the complex, orderly whole.

As I now know, it all started a very long time ago. I remember being horrified at a baby picture of me that looked like a grapefruit wearing a bonnet. I thought, "My God, I was fat and ugly even as a *baby.*" Apparently ignorance was to blame; while my mother worked, I was cared for by a succession of doting nurses who loved to stuff me with bananas. My resentment at being tampered with so early in life is irrelevant, since I kept on doing the same sort of thing to myself when I was old enough to make my own choices. My mother was away at work when I came home from school, and a sweet snack every afternoon was one of the most dependable comforts of my life. Thirty years later I still did most of my overeating then, though now it was my children coming home from school!

My childhood was happy, though in retrospect it is plain that all the seeds of my lifelong obsession with overweight were then unwittingly being sown. I was an only child, doted upon by my parents. Their willingness to grant my every wish confirmed my self-centered belief that the world existed for my pleasure alone, and that "me first" was an acceptable life motto. Indulgently, they gave me the sweets I constantly asked for, though clearly a chubby child would have been better off without them.

When I was grown, I read with a shock of recognition Jean Mayer's description of the inactivity that characterizes obese children. Hindsight shows me that as early as the third grade I had all the essential traits of the obese personality. As an only child, I was alone a good deal; I vastly preferred reading in my room to joining boisterous neighborhood games. On the school playground I didn't move as much or as fast as the thinner kids; I looked upon recess as a necessary evil, an interruption of my daily performance as teacher's pet. My last name then was McFadden, and (naturally) I was called McFatty. I didn't like it, but the teasing was on the whole good-natured.

In some ways my childhood was extremely joyous. I was a natural school leader; very outgoing and gregarious, I was school vice-president in fifth grade, school president in sixth. My fifth grade teacher wrote on my report card that I was an expert clown. I was not one of those withdrawn, disturbed, "weird" fat children everyone remembers from their school days; I functioned quite well among my peers. But all the life choices I continued to make on a daily basis tended in one direction only, as if I were assembling a giant jigsaw puzzle called Fat Person.

I still remember the horror of my first day in junior high school. I was still a plump gradeschooler, but I was now surrounded by *women* (many no older than myself), and I somehow knew even then that it was all over for me. I also remember my shame at having to line up with the other seventh grade girls wearing my new gym shorts that so embarrassingly revealed my chubby thighs. Before then I hadn't been aware of having "legs" or "thighs" in the adult sense, but I knew it now, and I could plainly see that mine didn't measure up.

Whatever personal equipment you were supposed to have, I didn't have it. I never again ran for a school office of any kind; I retreated desperately into the role of "brain" to salvage as much self-respect as I could in the face of my newly crippling social insecurities. There were now physical standards of performance, which I wanted desperately to meet but could not. (In retrospect, I'm glad I never learned how, since I would have willingly sacrificed anything to be thin, just like the driven, deluded victims of *anorexia nervosa* who starve themselves into emaciation—and sometimes death—today.) Three factors came together in a self-fulfilling whole: first, I was a perfectionist, who had always wanted to do well because that was how to please other people; second, newly sensitized, I had accepted wholeheartedly my culture's dictum that being fat was disgusting; third, I consequently found myself entirely unable to accept the particular woman's body I inhabited.

During this period I began my lifelong enslavement to diet articles and diet books. I had my first go with the Mayo Clinic Diet in tenth grade, followed in regular cycles by all the others that ever appeared. Each one took off anywhere from two to ten pounds, but each episode ended with my gaining the weight back. The term *yo-yo syndrome* hadn't been coined yet, but I was already a classic example of it. I fancied that people were always staring at me disapprovingly, and I practiced and embroidered defensive postures and rituals of camouflage. I seemed always to be clutching a coat in front of me. I despised having my picture taken, even in large family groups. I did not want any persistent evidence of the way I looked—a very strange attitude when you consider that *I* was the most persistent evidence of all!

I was never correctly proportioned for the clothes of the moment— the little bloomer bathing suits of the fifties, the miniskirt in the sixties, and so on. I lived very close to the beach, but I never sported a summer tan since I couldn't bear to be seen in a bathing suit. I used to own a disproportionate number of blouses. My fat was concentrated in my hips and thighs, and I always found it relatively less traumatic to try on clothing worn from the waist up—thus all the blouses. (Whenever I see an overweight woman with an elaborate, confectionlike coiffure, I think I understand her wish to beautify the most acceptable part of herself to the best of her ability.) I focused all my vanity on my waist, my best feature, and refused to wear any style, no matter how fashionable, that added any bulk whatever at the waist. I learned to sew, but that didn't help me much. My vanity extended to refusing to admit my actual hip measurements, so I once made myself a skirt that I could only wear standing up; I hadn't allowed enough width to permit sitting down. I believed that my body was out of proportion because of short arms and legs; sleeves and pant legs were always too long. I was in my thirties before I realized that my legs were exactly the right length for my pants when I wore small sizes—the problem had never been the length of my legs, but the circumference of my hips!

I didn't date much in high school. Looking back, I can see that the few boys I did date were wonderful people. But I was chronically dissatisfied with my dating "performance"; I was one of those people who, as Dr. Edward Stainbrook of the USC Medical Center once said in a lecture, "can't enjoy themselves simply because they aren't perfect." I can laugh now about one experience I had in high school, though it was terribly painful at the time. I was a sophomore, dating a wonderful senior I looked up to and adored. On what proved to be our last date, he observed that I would probably get along fine in life if I could ever learn to relax. I was crushed. Didn't he know that the only reason I held my stomach muscles in, tight as a drum, when we necked in the car was that I was afraid he wouldn't like me if he thought I was fat? I hadn't counted on being thought frigid when I was really only flab-conscious.

I did give great parties. I always pictured how much I could eat, then multiplied that amount by the number of guests. No one could eat those mounds of food—a double-edged situation, since when the guests didn't eat all the food at the party, there were scads of leftovers for the hostess to finish up afterward. Since I became aware of that aberration of mine, I notice it over and over: whenever fat people give parties, they always cook two or three times more food than their guests actually want to eat.

College was basically a replay of early adolescence, with a few variations. First, the fattening influence of starchy dorm food. (I still remember the hellishness of each college summer as I tried to take off the inevitable fifteen pounds I had put on in the course of the school year.) Second was emancipation from even minimal parental control and the delights of communal binging. (To teach us the social graces, teas were held in the dorms two afternoons a week; a few renegades like myself came to them regularly, but only to wolf down large numbers of cookies.) Added to the opportunities to binge almost constantly was the novel fact of having to be anxious about one's academic performance. Compulsive overeating in high school was never connected with my studies, but the academic pressures of college strengthened my tendency to overeat in response to anxiety. College also seemed to validate my silly idea that being an "intellectual" made it unnecessary to be athletic, an idea rejected by college girls today.

I still didn't date much, which I ascribed to my overwhelming unattractiveness. I wore timid clothes, never permitting myself to fantasize wearing, much less buying, anything really pretty, anything chic. I did have an ideal of chic, and I admired the girls who possessed it, but since I thought I couldn't possibly measure up, I considered it pointless even to try.

At the beginning of my senior year, however, the first fragmentary evidence of the "inner game" of losing weight appeared. At a party I unexpectedly met a man I knew instinctively I wanted to marry. I floated home in a daze, waiting for our date the following Saturday night. The next two weeks went by in the same way—thinking nothing but romantic thoughts about this dream man thirty miles away. My usual preoccupation with food and my weight vanished from my personal universe. I can still vividly remember getting on the scale in the dorm bathroom out of a sense of remote curiosity—only to find I had lost twenty pounds without being in the least aware of it! I was thunderstruck. This was so foreign to my notion of how one had to work at losing excess weight that it was as if a basic law of physics had been overturned. I had vaguely noticed my clothes had been getting looser, but now I looked more closely at myself and found I was actually a size 10! I couldn't believe it. Being in love was wonderful enough, but to be thin as well was a miracle. My joy was indescribable.

I stayed thin during the months that followed, which included our engagement and plans for marriage after my graduation from college. From the beginning, however, the marriage was not particularly happy. Both of us were graduate students, preoccupied with our separate anxieties. Soon I was regularly overeating again to make myself feel better, and soon after that I had ballooned to the point where I had only two dresses I could get into. (I still refused to entertain the notion of buying any clothes for a fat body I couldn't stand.)

My marriage thus provided me with a new rationale for overeating: the role of martyr. As long as I saw myself enduring innumerable discomforts for my husband's sake, it was imperative that I comfort myself some way. Naturally, my choice of comfort was food. My long commutes to my classes and back (more martyrdom) provided me with my first taste of a classic scenario: Eating in the Car. Eating in the car has only two minor problems: stop lights, when you have to pull alongside someone and they can see you eating, and disposal of the evidence when you get to your destination. This manner of eating and I were made for each other; I used it for practically the next fifteen years whenever I was driving anywhere alone. It isn't necessary to prolong the story of my first marriage, except to say that it was five years of uninterrupted "poor me." Overeating was how I made it up to myself for how miserable I was choosing to make myself feel.

When I finally summoned the courage to leave my husband, I discovered just how arbitrary my choice of the sad-sack role had been. I returned to California, to the most magical springtime of my life. I fell in love again, very unexpectedly, and once again out of sheer joy lost weight without conscious effort until I was again a size 10. I felt the most astonishing joie de vivre, which permeated every aspect of my life. The chronic moodiness that had characterized me ever since puberty vanished completely. My graduate studies were going well, and with my new sense of joy in my physical body I embarked on a physically demanding regime of a one-and-a-half-hour gym workout every day (which ordinarily would have been difficult for me even to contemplate). That summer I hiked all over the mountains of New Mexico, climbing 4,000 feet with ease, effortlessly keeping up with and sometimes even surpassing my male companion. I was thin and fit, and it was glorious!

Somewhat later I got my first real job and plunged into a large social group of co-workers interested in gourmet cooking. Under these circumstances, food was paradoxically not the problem it usually was. I forgot I had ever been droopy and dumpy and reveled in a new sense of attractiveness. For the first time in my life several men were attracted to me simultaneously. During this intensely exciting period I met the man who became my second husband two years later.

This marriage had everything my other marriage lacked. I loved my husband dearly and wanted to please him very much, but I found myself dogged by several familiar handicaps: moodiness, chronic tiredness, lack of enthusiasm. I had stopped working so I could finish my dissertation, and my bad eating habits had returned with a vengeance. Not only did I gain weight, but to my horror I found myself shuffling around the house crying a good part of every day. I had been intermittently moody since adolescence; the people close to me just came to accept this trait as something they had to put up with. I had always thought my moods were "justified"—understandable reactions to things that had happened (a bad grade, a personal rejection, etc.). But now I knew that something was wrong. I truly loved my new husband and my new life. None of my emotional problems was "real." I knew that the events in my life simply didn't justify feeling miserable, but I felt miserable just the same. In retrospect, I am thankful that the objective facts of my life at this time were obviously not the source of my misery. After all, I had a marvelous husband, I lived in my dream house, and so on. Because the problem *couldn't* be "out there," I was forced to look within for the source of the difficulty. If even one area of my life had been unpleasant or depressing (a "bad" husband, a boring job, an undesirable home, or difficult children), I probably would have blamed what were really *my* nutritional problems on external circumstances.

I thought I must be going crazy. I went to see a psychiatrist, who automatically prescribed antidepressant drugs, which I was reluctant to take. Soon afterward, George Watson's book *Nutrition and Your Mind* was published. I read it and was intrigued by its thesis about the relation of proper glucose metabolism to apparent neurosis and even psychosis. It explained in useful detail the fallacy of believing "moods" or neurotic episodes to be real. Instead, they are the inevitable result of a sugar-laden diet, which deranges the dependable supply of glucose to the brain. Junk food is not the path to clarity of mind. When the brain doesn't get the steady glucose it needs, it is capable of producing some rather bizarre thoughts and behavior, no less disturbing for being chimerical. I began to follow Dr. Watson's eating suggestions for my metabolic type and found that my depression vanished.

My story would be a success story that ended right here if I had been able to adhere to Dr. Watson's sensible eating plan for the rest of my life. But I wasn't, for I was one of those unfortunate people who are unable to bring themselves to do the right thing merely by knowing perfectly well what the right thing to do is. I continued my alternating cycle of dieting (self-pity) and binging (self-hatred) without interruption.

I gained thirty or so pounds with each of my two pregnancies. After the second I found to my dismay that my "base" weight (the weight around which my constantly fluctuating poundage tended to center) was higher than it had ever been. My gynecologist explained to me that each pregnancy makes a susceptible woman more carbohydrate-intolerant and thus more predisposed to diabetes than she was before. I thought, "Oh, no"; I didn't need another obstacle to losing weight. When I saw a diabetes checklist in the newspaper, I checked to see if I had any of the telltale warning symptoms. I had them all. My aesthetic objections to being fat were no longer my sole source of anxiety; now I could legitimately be apprehensive that my bad eating habits would sooner or later make me a diabetic.

At about this time a very curious event occurred in my life. I went with my husband on my first child-free vacation, a business trip to Atlanta followed by a vacation in Mexico City. I had a wonderful time—

sleeping late, shopping, pampering myself in general. By the time we came back I found I had lost ten pounds while eating everything I felt like eating. This was the most puzzling weight-loss episode of all; earlier I had decided that there indeed had been something magic about falling in love (a friend of mine had termed it the chemistry of rapture), but I didn't see how a simple vacation could produce the same wonderful effect. It was several years before I was able to put cause and effect together.

In January 1976 I read an article in *Vogue* about a new concept called the Protein Sparing Modified Fast (*The Last Chance Diet* did not appear for another ten months). A Los Angeles bariatrician (weight control specialist), Peter Lindner, was mentioned. I thought to myself, "This could do it; this could get me thin once and for all." The program of the Lindner Clinic was a very demanding, no-nonsense regime for very overweight people that consisted of a fast to ideal weight followed by two years of behavior modification therapy. The clinic was not interested in treating anyone who wanted anything less than to reduce to his or her ideal weight *for good*. Needless to say, I qualified. The first requirement was to adhere rigidly to a 1000-calorie diet for six weeks, writing down every bite we put in our mouths. I thought, "Impossible! I've never been able to stay on a diet longer than ten days at a time." But so intense was my desire to solve my problem once and for all, and so great was my hope that I had finally found the program that could do it, that I did the impossible, performing with virtual perfection. When the calorie counting was over and the fast began, we were required to visit the clinic daily for the first two weeks and three times a week thereafter. I did it without complaint—an eighty-mile round trip each time. Again, I was behaving impeccably; it pleased me to know my performance was as close to perfection as anyone could reasonably expect.

I fasted for six weeks and lost a total of thirty-nine pounds. When I had lost to within one pound of the goal weight the clinic had set for me, I skipped a menstrual period, a side effect that no one at the clinic could explain. Now I know the explanation: the fasting had caused me to stop producing estrogen, which temporarily stopped my periods. At the time, however, I panicked, convinced that I was pregnant and afraid that the fasting would damage the fetus.

I went home and began to overeat more senselessly than ever before in my life. Before I was always convinced that I overate because I *liked food*. Now I could see that this simply wasn't true. I ate anything—no matter how stale or tasteless or unappetizing—as long as it was made of carbohydrates. The more I ate, the more hysterical I became. All the hidden nightmares about myself were coming true, distressingly publicly. I gained twenty pounds the first two weeks, then lost most of it the next two. The "weight" I had lost came and went, over and over. The single lasting value of this horrendous experience was that it showed me clearly the distinction between gaining water weight and adding fat. Water filled my body, then flushed out again, in increments of ten pounds or more; meanwhile, the fat crept on inexorably, a millimeter at a time (it was like donning another wet suit each week). It took me three months to gain back all the pounds and inches that I had lost. All my co-workers, who had been so supportive and congratulatory as I lost my weight, now stood by and observed a tactful silence as I gained steadily. It was the closest to pure psychological torture that I ever hope to experience. I knew it was unfair. I had done everything anyone could be expected to do. Anything that was within the range of willpower to accomplish, I had shown I could accomplish. But this was a problem of an entirely different order.

I had never before been able to bring myself to admit that I *was* a compulsive overeater. Now, of course, I would have had to be a mental defective not to see the truth about myself. But even seeing that didn't help me any; I observed other people succeeding on various self-help programs but could never muster the ability to behave in a way that would have gotten me to my goal. My out-of-control behavior was still an enigma to me, since I was a person who believed so thoroughly in self-control and self-mastery in all other areas of my life.

A year or so later, I happened across Timothy Gallwey's book *Inner Tennis*. (I still marvel at how I came to read it, as I never have played and probably never will play tennis.) His concept of the Inner Game suddenly unlocked all the doors of my mind. I saw for the first time that my overeating was not a *sin*—it was merely a response, like a stroke in a tennis game. I could see clearly that all my attempts to lose weight had been dominated by my carping, self-critical, anxiety-ridden Self 1 to the point that my purposeful, goal-seeking Self 2 couldn't function at all. Falling in love and the trip to Atlanta were merely extraordinarily pleasant circumstances that allowed me to shed my chronic anxiety long enough for my body to take over and make me thin without conscious "trying."

Gallwey clarified all the issues for me. I still had lots of obstacles (ignorances) and personal resistances to overcome, but I did overcome them in the next year. About this time I came across Gregory Bateson's essay "The Cybernetics of Self: A Theory of Alcoholism" in his epochal book *Steps to an Ecology of Mind.* I joyfully realized that there was an intimate link between cybernetics and meditative experiences. As I said in Chapter 1, for an overeater who doesn't understand the sources of his behavior the world (not to mention himself) is of necessity irrational. For me it was a source of immense relief to understand the nature of my affliction and its relation to reality as a whole. For the first time I could entertain meaningful hope. I could see that I was responsible for the entirety of my predicament. I was not a victim; the problem was the result of my choice to spend my life being anxiety-ridden. Meditation (or happy, complimentary feedback, whichever way one wanted to look at it) was a successful way to rid myself of the anxiety, the most fundamental problem; learning new eating habits could then proceed with much less difficulty. I could see that "not-trying" was what was required. As the protagonist remarks in J. D. Salinger's *Zooey,* education should properly "begin [not] with a quest for knowledge at all but a quest, as Zen would put it, for no-knowledge."

I started seeing a highly gifted therapist named Susan Newton to learn more about how overeaters like me function. She taught me how arbitrary all our thoughts are: we can just as well choose to think supportive, constructive thoughts about ourselves as to think negative, carping thoughts. At one of our first sessions I burst out, "I wish I could stop thinking I'm so *ugly!*" I will never forget her soft reply: "If thinking you're ugly is the problem, and if thinking you're ugly resides in your mind, why did you think that losing weight would solve it?" She showed me that, given the way I was thinking, all the experiences in my life confirmed this prior self-diagnosis. At first, I couldn't understand this interpretation on any level but the intellectual; stuck in my habitual self-concept, I couldn't *feel* the truth of it. But help came from unexpected sources. One day I was sitting with my three-year-old daughter on my lap—as usual, thinking self-obsessed thoughts about being unattractive. My little girl suddenly looked up at me and said, "You're beautiful, Mama." It was a lovely moment.

To paraphrase the television program *That Was the Year That Was,* "There were two 1976s: the one that went on outside and the one that went on inside." When I focused on the latter, I began to see that the only significant reality for me consisted of inner events I had never paid attention to before. The outward events in my life existed in response to my inner life: the fixed emotional patterns I expressed. The events I have narrated are real—they actually happened—but their greater reality is showing how I worked at being "myself." My habituated emotions kept me perceiving myself and my world in the same old ways, which perpetuated my fixed emotions ad infinitum. Only by understanding that I had made that choice of pattern and then becoming willing to do something else instead could I hope to control my compulsive overeating. I couldn't become aware of this process as it was happening, but the pattern became clear in retrospect. The shibboleths that used to run my brain ("My bad moods are just *me*"; "I should get upset when I gain 'pounds' "; "I can't buy myself clothes until I can stand to look at myself in the dressing-room mirror") seem much less pressing now that I have my priorities sorted out.

My life now is focused on staying serene every day, willingly being disciplined in my behavior. It gives me a sense of satisfaction that overeating never provided in all my years of binging. People who have felt good all their lives may take it for granted. Not me. I *know* how wonderful it is to feel like this. I get to have every day be my birthday as long as I don't overeat. What else could I possibly want?

3
You Are Your Habits

My very chains and I grew friends,
So much a long communion tends
To make us what we are.

Byron, *The Prisoner of Chillon*

This chapter is not really about habits (as in what are called "bad eating habits"), but about the phenomenon of habituation and the way it impinges upon our ability to solve personal problems. What makes it especially difficult to understand ourselves as cybernetic entities is, as Gregory Bateson writes in *Steps to an Ecology of Mind,* that "the cybernetic nature of the self and the world tends to be imperceptible to consciousness." Nearly all of the goal-seeking activities of the organism take place subliminally, below the level of conscious awareness.

Why should nearly all of what is important to us happen below the level at which we can see what's going on? Evolutionary fitness: as Bateson explains, "No organism can afford to be conscious of matters with which it could deal at unconscious levels." In other words, any activity we repeat often enough *must* become automatic, for we would simply be unable to cope with having to "think" about innumerable activities, each consisting of innumerable small steps: driving a car, getting to the market, playing a piano piece from memory, and so on. Like computers, we have only so much present-moment processing capability; if we had to consciously think in order to perform everything we do, we wouldn't have any capacity left over to do anything new.

Everything we once learned to do, then chose to keep on doing, became an automatic part of us. First, we chose to perform the action (consciously); we repeated it (again by choice); it became habitual; it then became invisible to the conscious mind. Remember the old maxim "Practice makes perfect"; we all become more and more perfect (automatic and habitual) at doing the things we practice (repeat) many times. In fact, acquiring a habit can be thought of as acquiring a new skill. Bateson remarks, "The fact of skill indicates the presence of large unconscious components in the performance," and quotes Samuel Butler: "That which we know best is that of which we are least conscious." The brain simply does not need to pay attention to information it has already learned; automatic habits no longer send the brain any new information. After the organism's actions have become habitual, the brain will notice only if it does something *different* from what it is expected to do (a fact not without significance for dieters, as we shall see).

So far, our definition of *habits* seems to include only actions. However, thoughts and emotions can become habituated, too, and when they do, they also disappear from conscious awareness. Once our habitual ways of thinking and acting have become fully automatic, they become a part of our generalized definition of who we are. By this means they act to preserve us in our bodily equilibrium, a concept to be discussed in detail in the next chapter. In short, after we have decided who we are, our habits keep us predictably doing and being in the proper way; habituation keeps us from becoming someone entirely unrecognizable from one day to the next.

But as a servant of equilibrium (in other words, how things are now), habituation is clearly a natural enemy of *change*. A large inertia factor is built into our beings; as W. C. Ellerbroek writes, "We all tend to continue doing whatever we do." Our habits are the constituents of what makes us "feel right," which ensures that things will stay as close as possible to what we have already said we want them to be. E. H. Gombrich, an art historian, termed the brain a "continuity-monitoring" device. If something new and unexpected should occur, the brain would notice it immediately; all the novel sensory details of the experience would pour in, each one causing the brain to respond, "It's wrong. It's different. This isn't the way things ought to be." Think of making a turn onto a wrong street by mistake; long before you can verbalize what's gone wrong, you have a strong intuitive sense that something's amiss. All the usual habituated subliminal cues are missing, and the continuity-monitoring brain reacts. In international travel this temporary heightening of sensory receptivity is called culture shock. Foreign travelers almost always experience a hypersensitivity to any and all details of the alien environment—from the lettering on shop windows to the way table silver is arranged to minute peculiarities of idiom in a foreign language. Nothing is too trivial to escape remark, for everything is strange. After three weeks or so the traveler becomes habituated to the formerly strange place and settles down into a new definition of "things as they are."

The analogy may seem strange at first, but dieting as it is usually done is the equivalent of visiting a foreign country. By definition, all the foods you say you like (are used to) you don't get to eat; you make yourself stop your usual between-meal snacking; and you may even simultaneously start up an exercise program. All these new activities discombobulate your brain, for you're no longer doing any of the things that used to be "you." Everything you're doing represents new information, which (because it *is* new) needs to be noticed; therefore, much more sense data than usual is begging for attention from your conscious mind. All the salads and meager scoops of cottage cheese stand out in unappealing bold relief. And—as if that weren't enough—the fact that the brain is consciously noticing and processing this overload of sensory detail does a strange thing to your subjective sense of time: it slows it down considerably. It's like being on a drug trip that you would rather have skipped. For an achievement-oriented, impatient personality this maddeningly slow passage of time can be excruciating enough to justify giving it all up and sending out for a pizza.

The habituation and equilibrium functions are highly conservative; dieting is profoundly disturbing to both. A diet *is* a different way of doing things altogether. Not only does it entail a whole array of new and unfamiliar foods, but its ultimate aim is to make the body *itself* into something different, and nothing could possibly be more threatening to the body's equilibrium than that! No wonder the body sends up "danger" signals, trying its hardest to get the dieter to give up. The power struggle between the old order and the new makes most people so uncomfortable in the process that they do give up, then give themselves another black mark for "not having any will power." If you realize that a large part of you has been programmed to resist change at all costs, and that all the difficulties of the first few weeks are nothing more serious than the body's objections to having to form a new equilibrium, you will be less exasperated with yourself or impatient about your setbacks.

The truth is, much of the resistance we feel when we try to lose weight is the result of having chosen our methods poorly and having brought the wrong set of internal attitudes to the task. Your heightened perceptions and increased receptivity to suggestion at the beginning of any new experience are there to *help you learn it.* But you are the one who determines what you learn. Remember that the brain learns the state of mind connected with any experience as much as the experience itself; thus the brain is comprehending "disagreeable" as your reaction to diet food as much as the taste of the food itself. You're much better off if you can get your brain to process positive sensations, feelings, and states of mind as you do your learning on the path to your goal.

Disagreeable reactions to the unfamiliarity of any new experience are "learning jitters"—you feel uncomfortable simply because the new pattern has not arranged itself comfortably in the brain. In *Think Slim—Be Slim* Elyse Birkinshaw points out that resistance occurs inevitably when one's new programming encounters the old and that it is natural and to be expected (a comforting thought). As Dr. Laurence Reich says in *From Fat to Skinny,* "New activities are awkward the first time around. We tend to forget that initial period of awkwardness because, once learned, the behavior, skill, or whatever seems effortless."

If you ask people who have a remarkable skill, "How do you *do* that?" they're likely to reply, "I don't know; I just do it." To them, of course, it's habituated and effortless. I was always frustrated beyond words whenever I asked formerly fat acquaintances who were now thin "How did you *do* it?" and they answered, "I don't know" or simply, "I just stopped eating." Now I understand that they were telling me the truth as well as they understood it. Something in their lives had provided the initial impetus to change, and their bodyminds simply went about learning thinning behavior without the need for conscious attention to the problem.

Paradoxically, you are resisting learning if you continue to fill your conscious mind with anxious commentary about calorie values, scale readings, and your daily peccadilloes. This concentration on trivia makes your weight control efforts an entertaining, and deliberately perennial, pastime rather than a genuine attempt to change. When behavior is well and truly learned, it becomes automatic and invisible to the conscious mind; forcing your diet-related activities (and anxieties) to remain at the forefront of your conscious mind is a way of refusing to let good, disciplined behavior become automatic—and thus unremarkable to you.

The three-week changeover period mentioned earlier seems to be a minimum time required to adjust to and to automate new thoughts or new behavior. Various books (whether on bodies or minds) agree on this figure as the time necessary to learn new habits and discard the old. When asked whether his patients found his highly restrictive diets unpleasant, Nathan Pritikin replied (in *Family Circle* magazine), "It takes about 10 days to two weeks for tastes to change. The first to fourth days, you can't stand it. The second week, the food becomes palatable. The third week, you enjoy certain dishes. By the fourth week, you're saying: 'Delicious!' " Books on self-hypnosis usually recommend that any self-help suggestions be repeated daily for at least three weeks; in *Psycho-cybernetics* Maxwell Maltz claims that three weeks are required to effect a change in mental image.

It takes at least three weeks, then, for a new equilibrium to form itself out of a set of new habits presented to the body. But no dieter I've ever known (including myself, when I was a chronic dieter) has ever wanted a diet to last even that long. We define a diet as something you can *go off* at the end (if you don't quit before the end, that is). In other words, we understand a diet as something we *don't* want to learn to do automatically for the rest of our lives (given what some of us choose to eat while dieting, that's probably a good thing). I still remember how annoyed I felt whenever I read a book that stressed the point that good eating habits forever were what counted, not crash diets. I didn't want to hear that; I wanted the weight off now, all right, but frankly, pursuing "good eating habits" for the rest of my life sounded boring as hell. For that reason I sentenced myself to being on one diet after another for twenty-five years; all I practiced (repeated)—and therefore *all I learned to do*—was struggle and fail, over and over again.

It all boils down to the question, How permanent do you want this change to be? My answer to that would always have been, "I want to be thin for good," but my actions always ensured my being thin for about two days after the end of whatever diet I was on. The willingness to change, and thus ease of changing, operates on a sliding scale; we find it easiest to alter actions that have no particular emotional bearing on us. A road is rerouted; we don't argue, we merely make a new turn instantaneously. Someone once said to me, "Facts have a demand character." But other kinds of change come harder. As I said in Chapter 1, thanks to the thousands of books about diets and calories we all understand exactly what we should do; we all know that if we could lastingly change our bad habits we'd be guaranteed lifelong thinness. Dieters suffering from an excess of guilt often ask themselves rhetorically why it is they find themselves repeating behavior they *know* is bad for them. The only possible answer to this question is that it simply feels more comfortable than changing.

Every action you once elected to do had a purpose in your life. When it became automatic and habitual, the action continued intact whether the original reason for doing it still operated or not. I once read in a magazine article that whenever you do something out of habit you cannot be said to be choosing it. Once you become aware of what you are doing, you are choosing. A habit that's still in place out of simple inertia and unawareness, but which serves no present function in your life, is probably the easiest kind of all to discard; all that's needed is to become aware that you do it, then do it less and less until it disappears. Obviously, this kind of habit is very susceptible to treatment with behavior modification techniques. In *The Second Ring of Power* Carlos Castaneda quotes Don Juan's home-grown philosophy of how to dispose of unwanted habits with a minimum of discomfort:

"How can one stalk one's weaknesses, Gorda?"
"The same way you stalk prey. You figure out your routines until you know all the doing of your weaknesses and then you come upon them and pick them up like rabbits." . . . Don Juan had said that any habit was, in essence, a "doing," and that a doing needed all its parts in order to function. If some parts were missing, a doing was disassembled. . . . In other words, a habit needed all its component actions in order to be a live activity.

Behavior modification has become a highly popular tool in weight-management programs because it seems to work well. In *Fat and Thin: A Natural History of Obesity,* Anne Scott Beller remarks that "behavior therapy . . . outperform[s] other popular approaches by an impressive margin." Behavior modification is highly consistent with a cybernetic view of reality, since its major tools are awareness and feedback. Its premise is that all the actions we perform are learned; they have become habituated and thus invisible to us; when we become aware of them, we can substitute new behaviors in their place. With a suitable reward system we can be encouraged to learn the new behaviors to the point that *they* become automatic.

Behavior modification would undoubtedly be a hands-down winner in the competition among weight-loss strategies except for one small flaw. Behaviorists are the ultimate materialists; for them the only variables of importance are those which can be seen and measured (that is, the behavior itself). But it is becoming increasingly clear to those working in the field of brain physiology that behavior is merely the end point, the visible expression of a controlling *idea*. In *Steps to an Ecology of Mind* Bateson elucidates the distinction with great clarity: "The subject matter of cybernetics is not events and objects but the *information* 'carried' by events and objects."

Therefore, working to change specific actions may be an inefficient—even futile—approach if the source of the difficulty is some buried idea of unattractiveness, resentment, abandonment, or the like. In these cases the idea could be responsible for an entire collection of actions (which is why George Weinberg observes in *Self-Creation* that it may sometimes be easier to change a whole constellation of habits than to change just one). For example, when one feels unattractive as a result of being fat, the idea may be expressed in several disparate behaviors, such as folding one's arms over one's stomach for camouflage, buying dark-colored or timidly styled clothes, being reserved and shy with strangers, being hyperagreeable with friends and associates, wearing a coat in inappropriate weather, and so forth. It is not the behavior that is in any sense the source of the problem. Working at merely changing behavior without examining the controlling idea and trying to change *that* could have unexpected results; some new neurotic behavior could very well substitute for the old in expressing the controlling idea (as reformed alcoholics become smokers or ex-smokers become compulsive eaters).

But behavior modification techniques turn to their advantage an interesting fact about the human mind: deeply held ideas will sometimes change spontaneously merely as a result of practicing new behavior. This is the basis for the popular advice "act as if"—act as if you were slim, pretty, popular, and beautiful, and soon you will be so. Your habits belong to the person you say you are; conceivably if you change what you say you are, many of your habits will automatically adjust themselves. In other words, you acquire an idea, then you start to add behavior appropriate to that idea; soon your experiences "prove" to your subconscious mind that the idea must be true. As Joseph Chilton Pearce comments in *The Crack in the Cosmic Egg,* "We act ourselves into ways of believing and believe ourselves into ways of acting." I used to say that I was a shy person, so naturally in any social gathering I would act like one—withdrawn, never speaking until spoken to, and so on. I can't remember what made me change my mind about myself, but one day I did. For some reason I now tell myself that I am *not* a shy person, so now I go around having parties, greeting new neighbors, acting like an extrovert, and so forth. It would be impossible to say which is the "real me." Either one, of course, depending on what I say is so. In *Self-Creation* George Weinberg gives the theoretical basis for this phenomenon: "Every time you act, you add strength to the motivating idea behind what you've done." In fact, Weinberg goes so far as to claim we need to perform the acts in order to recharge the feelings; without the acts the idea would wither away.

Weinberg sees the self as entirely fluid, capable of changing in its entirety without great difficulty. "Nothing is frozen in your personality. . . . It's all subject to change." He claims that "people are, in effect, reinstating their personalities every day." He recommends that a person "sort through the continuous stream [of ideas] . . . and fish from that stream only those you want strengthened—and act on them." But Weinberg's hopeful outlook may be unrealistic with respect to certain classes of habituated actions. Earlier I gave the example of a rerouted road as an illustration of willingness to substitute new behavior for old instantaneously. Another example of this sort of willingness is suddenly becoming aware of behavior that used to serve a purpose but no longer does. What class do eating habits fall into? It depends on who you are. A few years ago my husband decided he wanted to weigh less than he did, so he promptly stopped eating a number of the starchy foods he was used to and, to my intense annoyance, lost thirty pounds fairly quickly. If he had been the gloating type (which he isn't), he could well have turned to me and said, "I did it. Why can't *you?*" Our situations were not parallel in any meaningful way. To my husband, who has no particular food attachments, food is simply nourishment; he's the kind that "eats to live." I, of course, have always been one who "lives to eat"; for me food has always been bound up with reward, comfort, festivity, the need to sustain feelings of adequacy, and more. I simply could not automatically summon up the same willingness that he did.

This leads to a definition of other classes of habits that are much harder to break than those discussed so far. While habits are merely unexamined behavior patterns, *compulsions* are habits fueled by an anxiety-producing habituated emotion or group of emotions. Even if the original cause of the emotion may have disappeared, the habituated emotion is still in place; consequently, the behavior which expresses it will be harder to get rid of. If it *is* extinguished, more than likely other types of compulsive behavior will spring up in its place.

The third class of habit is the most difficult of all to get rid of— that in which physiological habituation of the body is added to the habituated actions and emotions. This is called *addiction*. To be brutally frank, many overweight people are addicts, physiologically dependent on refined sugar. Because of the association of the word addiction with drugs, some fat people are simply unable to apply the label to themselves. I was one of these; I delayed seeking effective help for my problem for nine years because I could not bear to call myself a compulsive overeater.

Some habituation factors go beyond a single individual's actions, making it difficult if not impossible for him to change his own behavior or emotion. Everything connected with you forms a single habituated whole: your family, friends, job, home, and so on. If any of these relationships or environments puts pressure on you to continue eating (for example, your teenage children keep eating tempting food in your presence, or your husband criticizes you for being fat, which makes you anxious), you will undoubtedly continue to overeat.

Our culture also presents its members with an extraordinary assortment of double-binds. Gregory Bateson, who coined the term, defines a double-bind as a set of contradictory paths that punish you no matter which one you choose. A perfect example of a double-bind for an overweight female would be today's women's magazines, which feature alternating pages of luscious desserts and overly skinny models wearing the latest fashions. A double-bind will present you with anxiety no matter what your choice, and (as I will show in Chapter 5) anxiety is the basic source of all compulsive behavior. Eating as overweight people in our culture tend to do it is also a double-bind; at any given time most fat people are either dieting (in a spirit of self-pity) or binging (in a spirit of self-hate).

Habituated emotions are much more difficult to bring to conscious awareness than habituated actions. We all carry around in our brains messages to ourselves which have been repeated so often that we have become habituated to them; in other words, we don't hear them any more. Not being able to hear them doesn't mean that they aren't operating on us; on the contrary, they have already been encoded in our synapses and thus are truly part *of* us, not just something said *to* us. Becoming aware of our habituated thoughts and emotions is like asking fish to become aware of the water they swim in: it's invisible to them because it's so much *there*. Actions are at least visible; subliminal thoughts are not. Perception theory discusses *figure* (that which is perceived as a separate entity) and *ground* (that which is not differentiated). Habituated thoughts have become ground. Becoming aware of these messages is like turning up the volume on a faulty transistor radio: at first you get just a blur, then finally some sounds that make sense. My therapist Susan Newton once said to me, "Your mind keeps manufacturing in unlimited quantities any emotions you are still using." Neurologically speaking, it is probably more accurate to say that any emotion, once habituated, travels toward expression down well-worn neuron pathways that will continue as the path of least resistance until they are consciously altered in favor of some other emotion. But it is important to repeat that these habituated thoughts are indeed inaudible at first in order to make clear the distinction between them and one's usual conscious thoughts. Conscious thoughts can change from day to day, or moment to moment; you can feel happy one minute, sad the next. Habituated thoughts have worn a groove in the brain, so to speak; by now they have become the thoughts you can't choose to change or turn off.

One sort of habituated thought, more than any other, is responsible for all types of compulsive behavior: chronic anxiety. Chapter 6 presents a full-scale description of the biochemical basis of chronic low-grade anxiety; suffice it to say here that it represents a pervasive sense of worry about how things are going to turn out—and when. But chronic anxiety does not appear as such to the conscious mind. By definition our usual level of anxiety is invisible to us, so we call "anxiety" only a more severe attack of it. During the three months of my incredibly performance-oriented behavior at the Lindner Clinic I was just like a coiled spring inside, but I was totally unaware of it. I only noticed it—unavoidably—when it was transmuted into the binging that followed.

The definition of behavior modification earlier in this chapter was bringing to awareness the behavior to be changed, then learning new behavior to replace it. Behavior modification can work only in a climate of willingness. But often a person is not willing to look at the undesirable behavior and basically not willing to change it; this is resistance. Under these emotional circumstances habituation should more properly be called *repression*. As Dr. Theodore Isaac Rubin says in *Compassion and Self-Hate,* "We *repress* a great deal and in so doing are constantly engaging in the process of adding to the unconscious part of ourselves." We repress painful truths about ourselves in order to feel more comfortable than we would if we were conscious of them. Thaddeus Golas observed in *The Lazy Man's Guide to Enlightenment,* "What you cannot think about, you cannot control. What you cannot conceive of in your awareness, you will stumble over in your path." Golas says that if, by some perceptual quirk, we were unable to see automobiles, we would be in grave danger of constantly being run over by them; in the same way, we allow ourselves to be endangered by the consequences of our unexamined, repressed feelings.

As I said earlier, whatever you learn well becomes invisible and effortless. The only part of my former behavior that ever became invisible and effortless was my anxiety-ridden state of mind habitually connected with trying hard. As José Silva remarked in *The Silva Mind Control Method,* "If you think you want to give up a bad habit, chances are you are deceiving yourself. If you really wanted to give it up, it would fade away on its own. What you should want more than the habit itself is the benefit of giving it up. Once you learn to want the benefit strongly enough, you will become free of the 'unwanted' habit. Thinking about your habit and firmly resolving to give it up may bind you more tightly to it."

Chapter 7 will present a more detailed account of how you get from a resistant state of habituated anxious emotions to a state of awareness, willingness, and receptivity to change. At the moment the most important point to make concerns the wisdom of giving up the "dieting mind-set" as a way of bringing about lasting change. Of all human activities eating should become the most pleasurably effortless; the body is a complex machine designed to take care of your nourishment needs without further conscious intervention. Dieting intrudes officiously upon all these delicately balanced mechanisms, sometimes putting them out of commission altogether. Being thin is the body's accomplishment, one that it is basically willing to perform, given the right tools. This book will show you how your mind can help the body do its job rather than get in the way.

4
Bodymind

Your body is nothing more than your thought itself, in a
form you can see.
           Richard Bach, *Jonathan Livingston Seagull*

We need some entirely new ways to think about bodies, both our own
and others'. One of the most important ways is the notion—astonishing on the face of it—of giving up the attempt to control your weight
by struggle and will power and letting your body take care of the dieting.

We are firmly convinced that the body and mind are two separate
entities with very different roles. It's not entirely unreasonable to think
this; clearly, my mind cannot eat breakfast nor my body do algebra.
But the dichotomy is not the whole picture, either; it's closer to the
truth to say that the "body" and the "mind" represent two ends of a
continuum. We see the duality more clearly than the unity because of
the language we speak; as Dr. Edward Stainbrook so wittily put it,
"English is a marvelous language for nineteenth century physics; it
makes [discrete] states out of processes." Don Miller, the author of
Bodymind, says, "For convenience we call [the body and the mind]
separate things and think of them as opposites. But really they are
only the two poles of a single entity—which is the whole person." In
Zen Mind, Beginner's Mind Shunryu Suzuki gets to the heart of the
paradox: "Our body and mind are not two and not one. If you think
your body and mind are two, that is wrong; if you think that they are
one, that is also wrong. Our body and mind are both two *and* one."

Suzuki's statement is difficult to grasp. We can sense that we consist of *something* beyond what we hear to be our conscious mind and
what we see to be our body, though we hesitate to think this "something" is either a species of mind (because it can't talk) or a species of

body (because it's not visible). Many names have been used to label it: the subconscious mind, the universal self, a higher power, the thinking body, Self 2, and so forth. In Michael Murphy's *Golf in the Kingdom* it is called the "inner body" and described (echoing the cyberneticist Norbert Wiener) as "not bound to the physical frame it inhabits. It is far more elastic and free, more like a flame than a rock." Like Ken Dychtwald or Don Miller, I use the term *bodymind* to refer to this elusive entity—our personal, ongoing biofeedback learning system.

In *Mind as Healer, Mind as Slayer* Kenneth Pelletier says, "The neurological evidence suggests a dialogue between autonomic processes and the centers of thought in the cerebral cortex. The reticular [activating] system is one of the best pieces of neurophysiological evidence for a profound interconnection between mind and body." The results of reticular system activity are found everywhere; the placebo effect, for example, is a well known and frequently repeated instance of it. Experimental evidence for the link is mounting rapidly. (In one study, cited in Pearce's *Crack in the Cosmic Egg,* hypnotized hungry people were told they had eaten, and their blood sugar levels promptly rose.) An entirely new biological world view is shaping itself. In *Eating Disorders* Hilde Bruch writes, "With recognition of the inadequacy of the mechanistic model for understanding of major areas of biological and psychological facts, a great shift in the life sciences has come about. There is less concern with the transmission of *energy;* the movement is toward models in which it is transmission of *information* and *meaning* that matters most."

Don Miller observes, "There's no bodily event that goes unregistered in the mind, and no mental occurrence that doesn't affect your body in some way. The healthier you become, the more 'together' your mind and body get to be—until finally they form a single united entity, the bodymind of the whole person." It's like two people wearing a horse costume; they simply can't do anything unless they can agree about what direction *both* of them are going to walk.

One of our most damaging cultural blind spots is the failure to grasp the immense significance of both body-mind unity and the nonverbal cognitive abilities called visceral learning. It's understandable that we should identify with our conscious mind: because it can talk, it seems to be the "smart" part of us. But it has never occurred to us that the chattering part of ourself could be like a performer taking its cue from some higher, more intelligent source. We think the conscious mind *must* be prior because it is aware of the body, not vice versa. This chapter will argue that both our visible body and the functions we think are controlled by the conscious mind (such as our food preferences) are really the responsibility of the bodymind, which comprehends both.

Let us examine the reciprocal processes by which any body is created. Carl Frederick has used the startling description, "Your body is simply a living expression of your point-of-view about the world." To think of a solid object as an expression of a point of view requires a mental leap most of us are not accustomed to making. Listen to it again, this time from Peter Caddy, the founder of Findhorn, the New Age spiritual community located in Northern Scotland. In Paul Hawken's *The Magic of Findhorn,* Caddy complains that when one shows most people a prodigious cabbage such as those grown at Findhorn, they "think only in terms of size, form, and quantity. They take for granted the being and consciousness behind that [forty-pound] cabbage." *Being* and *consciousness,* intangibles both, impinge upon (indeed, create) the tangible reality we in the Western world are so fascinated with.

In *Your Body Speaks Its Mind* Stanley Keleman remarks, "Our bodies are us as process, not us as thing. Structure is slowed-down process." Everyone's body consists of a long series of choices made according to some antecedent definition of identity; the idea is prior to its realization in time and space. The bodymind's task is the continual processing of transactions and messages, whether using the semantics of spoken language or of neurohormones. One's extra pounds are nothing but the cumulative result of thousands of problem-solving transactions. Susan Newton once told me that overweight should be thought of not as a problem so much as a solution to something (a notion echoed by Hilde Bruch in *Eating Disorders*). Susan had me repeat an affirmation that began, "I create my body from moment to moment." Yes; we *must* create our body from moment to moment or it would ultimately disappear; eating is the continual process of replenishment by which the body remains visible. Each and every body's natural and normal state is health; any overweight person is that way because of having created some obstacles that prevent the body from returning to a healthy state.

Frequently, however, those obstacles seem utterly insurmountable. One well-known axiom any dieter would agree with is that it is hard to change your weight at all, and even harder to change it for good. This fact is simply a function of body equilibrium or, in biological terminology, *homeostasis*. As Anne Scott Beller says in *Fat and Thin*, "The immutability of the equation between excess calories ingested and the weight that is automatically supposed to accrue from them may prove on second thought to be subject to a wide range of empirical ifs, ands, and buts. Human metabolism, commonly assumed to be an absolutely unvarying example of the laws of thermodynamics in action, has proved upon closer examination to be subject to a wide range of variation among individuals." It's something of a relief to hear this, actually; dieters have long been mentally tortured by moralizing doctors lecturing them on the energy balance theory: calories in versus calories out equals your weight. Recent research has definitely shown the body's resistance to change (either up or down) to be more pervasive than was ever thought. Beller reports, "Investigators doing closely controlled clinical studies have found that, depending on metabolic factors that vary at random from one subject to the next, it can take anywhere from a low of 1,250 to a high of 3,000 calories to add a pound of fat to the patient's own pre-experimental weight."

Dr. Lindner once told me an anecdote about a patient who came to him to gain weight. All of her body functions consistently tested as normal, but nothing could make her gain. In desperation, after nothing he did seemed to help, Dr. Lindner put his patient on a regime of 5,000 calories a day and complete bed rest. She still didn't gain anything! The energy-balance theory may cover a lot of ground, but it still doesn't adequately explain cases of this type at both ends of the metabolic spectrum. The notion that the bodymind's homeostasis is mutually reinforced by metabolic conditions and fixed mental patterns does a lot to explain why body equilibrium should be so resistant to our most earnest efforts at adjustment.

Homeostasis is indeed a biological miracle, but it's safe to say that fat people see it as an unmitigated disaster. Further, for most obese people, body-mind unity—the fact of being intimately bound up in and with a recalcitrant body—is a tragic mistake, a source of daily horror. The overweight person's bad relationship with his or her body is just like a bad marriage without hope of divorce: being forced to live on close terms with someone you're ashamed of and whose actions you deplore, wishing you could be anywhere but where you are. As Alexander Lowen writes in *The Betrayal of the Body,*

A body is forsaken when it becomes a source of pain and humiliation instead of pleasure and pride. Under these conditions the person refuses to accept or identify with his body. He turns against it. . . . He may attempt to transform it into a more desirable object . . . but it will never provide the joy and satisfaction that the "alive" body offers. . . . People are so accustomed to thinking of the body as an instrument or a tool of the mind that they accept its relative deadness as a normal state. They measure bodies in pounds and inches, and compare their shape with idealized forms, completely ignoring the fact that what is important is how the body feels.

Since almost all our activities in this culture are thought of as performances, it was inevitable that bodies came to be included in this generalized performance valuation. One's body is highly visible; its shape and decoration are the constituents of sex appeal, and as such it is clearly susceptible to being judged according to performance criteria. We have very strong ideas about, and very stringent criteria for, what bodies should look like in order to be acceptable, and even stronger ideas about what deviations are considered simply unacceptable. One issue of *Ms.* magazine, discussing "the politics of body image," concluded that in this country nearly all women—no matter how close to the physical ideal—are made to feel dissatisfaction with their bodies.

The only trouble is that one's body is emphatically *not* a performance. It is a visible expression of the state of one's entire being. I failed over and over in my weight-loss attempts because I was trying to change my body, when what really needed changing was the inner me; after I had changed that, my body improved spontaneously. Oscar Ichazo, the founder of the Arica system for personal development, discusses the problems attendant upon seeing the body as a performance and trying to alter its functioning according to some prior mental definition of acceptability:

An imbalance occurs in our lives because our body and our psyche work in constant opposition to each other. The physical body has its own limitations; it is subject to rules for the maintenance of health and to all the physical laws which govern its development. . . . The aims and aspirations of the psyche oppose those of the body. In the normal human being a permanent contradiction exists between the ambitions of the psyche and the limitations of the body.

Obese people are those who simply cannot accept either their body's beauty or its competence. R. D. Laing claims in *The Divided*

Self that people like this have lost their "sense of basic unity" because they "have come to experience themselves as primarily split into a mind and a body. Usually they feel most closely identified with the 'mind'." Actually, they can't be blamed for trusting their minds instead of their bodies, since their bodies have never seemed worthy of trust. The fat person's life problems center upon his or her body and its malfunctions. A fat person's mind often malfunctions, too—depression, chronic anxiety, and so forth—but since no one has thought to look at the mind as a reflection of the body's state of health, only a few physicians, and almost no psychiatrists, understand that many neurotic emotions simply go away when the body recovers its health. Most normal, instinctual body functions have been damaged in an overweight person. Don Miller says,

Every living creature is equipped by nature with a *food instinct*—a built-in, unconscious mechanism that tells the animal what things are food and what things are not food. . . . The human animal is also equipped with a food instinct—only it is distorted, buried, deflected, even destroyed by our culture, with its strange faith in thinking as *the* solution to all of our problems—and its rejection, suppression, and mistrust of all that is instinctual, sensual, and animal in human nature.

The food instinct normally called *hunger* has been replaced by stress-initiated food cravings which cannot be sated. You think you "have" food preferences; food cravings, on the other hand, "have" you.

I still remember the first book on food awareness I ever read, Leonard and Lillian Pearson's *The Psychologist's Eat-Anything Diet Book.* The book makes the distinction between foods that "hum" to you (the foods you *really* want, deep down inside) and foods that only "beckon" to you (tempt you as you pass by them). The Pearsons' point is that fat people never let themselves have the food they really want (because they define it as sinful) and therefore spend the rest of their lives overeating as a compensation for this deprivation. The awareness exercises in the book are designed to help the reader identify which foods "hum" and those which merely "beckon," in order to cut out the latter and concentrate on the former. I was reluctant to do the exercises, since I thought I adored every high-calorie food known, and I knew I'd end up with a list of a hundred or more "humming" foods. But I was wrong. I conscientiously did the exercises and found that, on the contrary, *no* foods hummed to me. Since I didn't understand allergy addiction at the time, it was a puzzling, almost nonsensical, find-ing; I was still binging out of control on all the foods that the tests told me I didn't really care for. Now, of course, I know that the tests told the truth; for me those foods I "loved" did not function as food but es-sentially as narcotics. In *The Compulsive Overeater* George Christians wryly remarks, "I never heard of a compulsive eater who *ever* felt full. Bloated, yes. Ready to vomit, yes. Sweating and gagging, yes. But 'full'—never!"

Irrationality like this leads the fat person to conclude that the body is wayward and needs to be rigidly controlled to prevent it from fur-ther shaming its owner. As Chapter 8 explains, fat people are usually terrified of the idea of giving up control over themselves; they think of it as the equivalent of letting a mental incompetent hold a responsible job—who knows what disaster would follow? Their rational mind, schooled to control, cannot comprehend that the irrational things the body seems to be doing are simply the things it *must* do, given the cir-cumstances. The major source of the difficulty is the failure to under-stand the body rather than leap to moral judgments about what it "should" be doing.

As I remarked earlier, a chronic dieter's life is based on several un-pleasant realities: a disheartening lack of overall progress in spite of repetitively losing and gaining over and over again. It's the worst of both worlds—always being on the way, then waylaid by cravings, nev-er achieving the goal permanently. In *Forever Thin* Dr. Theodore Isaac Rubin sagely identifies the *entire* performance, both gaining and losing, as a single cycle:

What looks like a history of repeated victory and failure is actually no such thing at all. These cycles or phases are simply part and parcel of the obese profile in which insight and real control on a sustained level are utterly lack-ing.... Doctors, therapists, and commercial weight-reduction groups often take undue credit for an obese person's weight loss when in fact they have only happened to "treat" him in his thinning phase—which inevitably passes on to a fat phase again.

Performance-oriented dieters like to lose and hate to gain, but they are resolutely unaware that, given all their life choices, the one implies the other. I remember once becoming dimly conscious that on the whole I spent about half of each month dieting and the other half binging, but I did not yet understand that *each made the other necessary* to preserve my peculiar equilibrium. In *Thin Forever* Dr. Alberto Cormillot observes, "The fat person is ill, but he nevertheless maintains a balance—not the best possible one, but the least harmful one. Every human being, at every moment of his life, places himself in the *least harmful* situation possible."

Addiction (including carbohydrate addiction) provides a similar compensating balance. As Stanton Peele and Archie Brodsky's *Love and Addiction* explains, "A person repeatedly seeks artificial infusion of a sensation, whether it be one of somnolence or vitality, that is not supplied by the organic balance of his life as a whole." Chapter 6 will go into much greater detail about the way in which chronically anxious people—such as I was—set up a bodily imbalance which requires redress by the temporary calming effect of sugar and consequent release of insulin. The addiction itself is thus not a disturbance, but a symptom of and a compensation for a prior disturbance or malfunction.

The body carries out innumerable unseen activities just to keep each person in equilibrium. The body is a miracle, performing each day a wide range of extremely complex functions over a range of conditions that would cause other, lesser machines to sputter and die. Each of the body's crucial mechanisms (breathing, cooling itself, transporting water, and so forth) has at least five "fail-safe" mechanisms or alternate pathways by which the function can be accomplished, which ensures that the body won't fail even if component parts do. We need to talk about all the fail-safe mechanisms because it is essential that every dieter be impressed with this one fact about the body: it is going to do what it has to do, come hell or high water.

As we've all been told many times before, we would find it utterly impossible to perform even a simple act like walking down the street if we had to direct each movement consciously. It is just as silly and futile to try to control the operation of our bodies—but this one is apparently harder to see. We have become accustomed to thinking of our bodies as helpless children needing our constant attention and direction, though a more foolish attitude could scarcely be imagined. It is in fact physiologically impossible to "control" your body while on a diet, though everyone in our culture seems to agree that this is exactly what should be done. As I see it, trying to control your body is very much like trying to pass by a large, playful dog: the harder you push, trying to get by, the more it thinks you want to play and the harder it leaps at you. So the first reason to give up trying to control your body is that doing so will make you anxious and nervous, which is not good for you. The second, more important, reason is that it simply *will not work.*

Diets as we know them are diabolical schemes for keeping over-weight people estranged from their bodies. Every month or so a "new" one comes out in a newspaper or magazine. You cut out the diet and decide to have a go at it. (This is like seeing a size 4 pair of shoes in a shop window and buying them even though your feet are a size 8.) When you're on the diet, you're so obsessed with performing well on it, following all the instructions, that you can't be bothered to notice what your body is trying to tell you—until it starts talking quite loudly and insistently (you faint, or feel lightheaded, or get terribly grouchy). You go off the diet and blame yourself for your "lack of will power." Grant Gwinup's *Energetics,* a best-selling diet book of a few years ago, repeatedly made the point that the body's need to establish and maintain its equilibrium by balancing overall food intake would always play havoc with a dieter's best-laid plans: "Our appetites not only tell us when to eat and how much to eat, but also what proportion of carbohydrate, fat, and protein to eat. . . . It is also fortunate that when one of our medical interns occasionally prescribes a diet which is—by mistake—terribly out of balance, no harm is really done, because the patient won't follow it very long. . . . The average person will stick to [a fad diet] for about three days."

The problem is not the dieter's lack of factual knowledge about calories, carbohydrate grams, and such, but a basic lack of respect for the body's inner wisdom. Everything your body tells you—as unacceptable as the message may be—makes sense; everything it says has a reason. Ignoring the message, or trying to muffle it or change it, is simply a willful ignoring of the clearest form of reality you have access to. You may not like your overweight body very much, or like what it is saying, but it is being as honest with you as it can at the moment. Every one of its infirmities speaks of the wish to return to health.

The overweight person's continual attempts to force "good behavior" on an unhealthy body is like having broken your leg and then forcing yourself to do your daily jogging (cursing your malperforming leg all the while) instead of simply attending to your injury. When your body misbehaves, it's because it is in trouble. First it needs to be healed, then it will do what you want it to do naturally and effortlessly.

In *The Lives of a Cell* and *The Medusa and the Snail* Dr. Lewis

Thomas returns again and again to the theme of the aesthetic complexity of the natural world and the human organism. Reading Dr. Thomas, one is struck forcibly by his eloquent tales of the intricate beauty available to the biologist's perusal—the orderly minutiae at all levels of all living things. Awed by the majesty of the large and the small, how could we have the temerity to think we need step in and direct it?

Timothy Gallwey's books are mostly about sports, but *Inner Tennis* contains a brief subsection describing his middle-aged tennis pupil Molly's attempt to apply Gallwey's principles to losing weight. She decided simply to go to the grocery store and buy only what her body told her it wanted to eat, with no preconceptions or prejudices. As she reported to Gallwey, for three weeks her body told her to eat cabbage and more cabbage. Since she had never particularly cared for cabbage before, she found this rather strange, but she did it anyway—and lost fifteen pounds. The body's apparently arbitrary recommendation of cabbage was actually impeccable bariatric medicine. Molly probably had an excess of sodium in her body and thus was retaining water. Eating the potassium-rich, low-calorie cabbage put her body in better acid-alkaline balance, eliminating both the water she had been retaining and some fat as well. Not every overweight person will hear such clear messages of health right from the beginning, as later chapters will explain. Sometimes the body has to become healthier before the messages are this clear and coherent. But as Don Gerrard, the author of *One Bowl,* reminds us, "Nowhere are we taught that our bodies can regulate themselves, or heal themselves. And we are not taught that our inner feelings and sensations are the signals by which this regulation or this healing is effected. On the contrary, we have been taught to ignore these *inner* signals, which come from ourselves, in favor of listening to various *outer* authorities, experts and specialists."

So far this chapter may have seemed slightly schizophrenic, detailing all the ways the fat person's body lets him down, yet insisting that the only sane way to proceed is to listen to the body rather than try to control it by force. It is now time to resolve the apparent contradiction by looking at the problem as an issue of language comprehension.

The biggest obstacle to reading the body's messages is that we've lost the key to understanding what it's saying. It's very much as if the body were speaking highly rhetorical classical Greek, but because we didn't understand Greek, we took it to be spouting gibberish. Or perhaps it's better described as an issue of mistranslation. The body's language, like classical Greek, is *archaic*: our food needs were defined several million years ago, long before the invention of processed food. Therefore, there may be an immense gulf between the food or substance the body is actually requesting and what we in our ignorance select to eat.

Take, for example, the perennial human "sweet tooth," the bane of a fat person's existence. The question is logical: why do we even *have* a sweet tooth if we weren't meant to be eating Twinkies? Well, from the point of view of the archaic body, we can hypothesize that the inborn predilection for sweetness is intended as a pointer to sources of vitamin C. Millions of years ago—through what may have been an evolutionary fluke—human beings lost the ability to synthesize their own vitamin C. Since vitamin C is vital to stress management in the body, humans had to develop a craving that would lead them to seek out the fruits which were its richest source. Similarly, our inborn taste for salt probably exists because millions of years ago we were largely herbivorous and (like deer) needed salt to balance the overload of potassium our vegetarian diet provided. All these cravings do exist in the body, and they once had a life-enhancing function. Now, however, food manufacturers capitalize on them, increasing their profits by giving us too much of "what we want"—more concentrated sources of salt and sugar than we were ever intended to have—and we suffer accordingly.

The mistranslation problem and its ramifications cover much, but not all, of the ground. Undeniably, some of the messages sent by an unhealthy body are pathological (for instance, the sudden gain of large amounts of weight, constant cravings for sweets, and continual hunger), and it is these that alarm the fat person into thinking his or her body is undisciplined and must be ruled with an iron will.

But let us again look at it as a language problem, this time considering the potential usefulness of communications with little or no semantic coherence. If someone streaked by you babbling hysterically, you wouldn't need the message to be grammatically perfect to know that something was wrong. The body's incoherent messages are symptoms—a "strong demand for change," as Hal Bennett and Mike Samuels, the authors of *Be Well,* so nicely phrase it. In our culture we prefer to mask symptoms rather than deal with their underlying causes. Similarly, if we insist on seeing our weight loss efforts as a "performance," when the body asserts its needs, we are likely to be annoyed at the inconvenient lack of "results" rather than attentive to the contents of the message.

We still face the contradiction that (a) it is our body's misbehavior that makes us want to take over control, but (b) control is absolutely the wrong strategy for solving the problem. The inappropriate tendency toward overcontrol is like someone wanting to play golf on a tennis court—an example of utter insensitivity to the real dimensions of the situation. A book on food awareness like *The Psychologist's Eat-Anything Diet Book* is very useful for showing us the arbitrariness of our culturally determined food behavior, such as our insistence on "balanced meals" three times a day, and so on. With our rigid definitions we may be totally insensitive to the reality of the body's food-need cycles; it could be that we don't need to "balance" our food intake every day, but only every week or so. In *Eating is Okay!* Dr. Henry A. Jordan says, "[Some patients] say the trouble is that they 'go on binges.' Binge? What's a binge? ... Most people who tell us they've been on binges are simply feeling guilty because of eating a little extra food some night." One day I realized that all the emphasis on how much food a dieter should eat at one sitting was completely irrelevant; the only thing that mattered was to wait until really hungry before eating again (if you had eaten a lot, the wait would simply be longer). This strategy cannot be used by people who are not yet in a healthy equilibrium, however. Because their metabolism is governed by chronic stress, they cannot perceive true hunger signals, for the lowered blood sugar that results from excessive insulin output continually provides a false sense of hunger—which is why, incidentally, hypoglycemia is called the "hunger disease."

Perhaps a better understanding of the nature of homeostasis, and the difference between normal and deranged equilibrium, will help us to appreciate the body's majesty and complexity. As Norbert Wiener observed in *Cybernetics,* "Our inner economy must contain an assembly of thermostats, automatic hydrogen-ion-concentration controls, governors, and the like, which would be adequate for a great chemical plant. These are what we know collectively as our homeostatic mechanism."

The body is a goal-seeking mechanism, and homeostasis is the process by which it achieves its goal, the continuation of life. Homeostasis is a powerful force to keep us the same in the face of constant cellular change. The body's operation is governed by a constant exchange of feedback. Elsewhere in this book the term *feedback* seems synonymous with "thoughts" or "mental suggestions," but here it is used in its more elemental sense: the body is a feedback-governed *engine*. Feedback is responsible for starting and stopping or adjusting actual physiological processes: hormone flow, heart rate, and so forth.

In the context of homeostasis, we say that the body is a *stable oscillating system*. This seemingly paradoxical phrase is just as significant as Suzuki's "not two and not one"; it is necessary to understand both that the body is stable in the long term and that its stability consists of short-term self-corrective oscillations. According to W. Ross Ashby's *Design for a Brain*, "Every stable system has the property that if displaced from a state of equilibrium and released, the subsequent movement is so matched to the initial displacement that the system is brought back to the state of equilibrium."

We also need to introduce the concept of *sensitivity*, which means almost the opposite of what we have in mind when we say someone is "sensitive" (that is, oversensitive, reacting excessively to every little event). A highly sensitive closed-loop feedback system is one characterized by very small reactions: it is capable of detecting tiny changes and compensating for them immediately, which makes large-scale fluctuations or changes of state unnecessary.

A person in good health, eating the right kinds of food, will have a sensitive body whose weight does not fluctuate much. (We all know people who claim that their weight has not varied by more than a pound or so in twenty years.) These are people who can trust their food instincts; they are not interested in eating unless they are hungry, and when they *are* hungry they listen to their bodies and are guided to the right food to eat. Sometimes the large amounts they eat, seemingly without punishment, make a self-depriving dieter blanch. I have been an example of both types in my life: I was once a person who could put on two or three pounds after a single ill-advised meal; now that my body is healthier, my weight has not fluctuated by more than two pounds for nearly a year.

The bodymind is rhythmic and periodical in everything it does, though only a few of its cycles (such as the menstrual cycle) are obvious to the casual observer. Dr. Ronald Gatty, in *The Body Clock Diet*, states that if a hungry person were to postpone eating for even a few minutes, the desire would probably wane, since we are all on a ninety-minute cycle of alternating hunger and satiety. (Stanley Keleman's observation that life seems to consist of alternating cycles of excitement and rest is borne out on every bodily level down to the neuron, whose alternation of firing and rest comprises the most fundamental activity of our beings.)

Unfortunately, our goal-striving minds are not cyclical, but linear, obsessed with "results." In the twentieth century we have become accustomed to being the masters of machines whose speed we can control. The body, however, is a primitive engine whose speed we *cannot* control—and we find this fact highly frustrating. We want our body's weight loss progress to be steady, and to occur at an unrealistic rate of speed. Whenever the body fails to comply, we feel anxious, unaware that this response is in itself a significant barrier to progress.

What the overweight person sees as the body's irrational behavior is nothing but the exaggerated cycles characteristic of an insensitive, deranged system. The stability of a deranged system consists of a continuing series of instabilities, like a Charlie Chaplin tightrope act: veering from one near-disaster to another. In *Body, Mind, and Sugar* Abrahamson and Pezet compare body stability to driving a car (whether well or poorly). The most efficient way to drive a car down the street is to make very small corrections with the steering wheel, mostly progressing straight ahead. Some idiosyncratic drivers drive by flinging the steering wheel from one side to the other, making the car careen from side to side. It's still forward locomotion, but it's highly unstable and no one would recommend it as the proper approach.

The large oscillations that characterize a body in an unhealthy equilibrium are primarily due to the ramifications of the stress response. Later chapters will discuss the stress response in more detail; in this chapter we are interested only in the way in which unwise eating initiates it. The stress response is basically a homeostatic mechanism called into play when the body is threatened by something, to try to restore balance. It can be elicited to neutralize the effects of toxic food on the body. But here's the paradox: the stress response *itself* can be deleterious. It's like the combination of poison and antidote: you'd have been better off with neither.

We talk a lot, dutifully, about eating "food that is good for us," implying that our truer preferences would be junk food. What *is* "good for us"? What does *toxic* mean? All food exists somewhere on a sliding scale between being downright poisonous to us (that is, so toxic that the body can't manage it at all) and agreeing with us perfectly. Allergens are toxic to some people but innocuous to others. The "best" (least toxic) food is that which can be digested without eliciting the stress response (it's not poisonous, we're not allergic to it). The foods we all tend to tolerate best are those that are closest to the body's natural acid-alkaline balance (pH) and that contain substances required by the digestive process—in other words, food as close as possible to its natural state. When we eat food that has been stripped of its vitamins, enzymes, and fiber content by overprocessing, its natural pH or digestibility changed by the addition of sugar, salt, preservatives, and colorants, the body may react with the stress response (its magnitude depending on how much the food has been altered). For example, to be digested properly, the carbohydrates in your food require three times their weight in water. Fruits already contain enough water to balance their carbohydrate content; products made of refined sugar probably do not (a piece of fruit typically contains 20 grams of carbohydrate, a piece of cake closer to 75). Eating concentrated carbohydrates stresses the body; the deleterious effects of the stress response (edema, excess insulin output) follow, giving rise to large weight fluctuations and disturbances in other functions.

It should be obvious by now that the long-term solution to anyone's weight problem is not more baroque eating regimes or torturous behavior-altering schemes; a better goal is to remove stress from the mind (through relaxation) and the body (through healthy food), and then to eat according to the body's needs and on its schedule.

Biofeedback is a discipline that is just now coming into its own. Before the first nearly accidental discoveries were made, no one considered that the body's autonomic systems were educatable. But they quite clearly are, and by a route diametrically opposed to what we have always called "education" (since we have always equated education with control). As Barbara Brown, the biofeedback expert, observed in an interview, biofeedback "is basically a process of 'letting it happen' or of 'letting go' of conscious and subconscious control. . . . The ability to learn control over body functions is inherent in human beings although little used because of inhibitions generated by educational and medical traditions."

As Chapter 12 will discuss in detail, learning how to direct your bodymind without trying to usurp control may be merely a matter of learning to issue clear instructions. If typical best-selling diet books are any indication, we don't understand the principle of giving unambiguous directions at all well. Someone who sincerely wants to weigh less but also sincerely wants to be allowed to eat like a pig cannot be said to be issuing clear instructions to the bodymind. Behavior modification specialists will tell you that the most effective learning situation is one in which you do something and then get rewarded. The trouble is that if you have defined the only satisfying reward as one that contradicts the basic laws of human physiology, you're in for a little trouble.

Whenever you set out to learn something, you need to channel a majority of your effort into overcoming the resistance of the first three weeks or so, for it's then that the bodymind's inertia (its devotion to the way things "used to be") is at its height. In *Fat and Thin* Anne Scott Beller quotes a psychologist as saying that overweight people tend to be at a particular disadvantage in situations that require abandoning one response and developing a new one. Starting up any self-improvement project (losing weight in particular) is like sending off a rocket to the moon: we need to accept the fact that a huge commitment of energy will be needed at first just to get into orbit; after that the effort required diminishes markedly.

As I've said several times before, a workable body-mind relationship is difficult to maintain unless the body is healthy. Chapter 14 provides step-by-step instructions about how to get that way. A better mental state is one of the products of the body's health; as Bennett and Samuels write in *Be Well,* "Feelings of ease and dis-ease probably always involve both body and mind. . . . A feeling of ease might include a tranquil state of mind along with relaxed muscles throughout your body." We need to constantly keep in mind the reciprocal feedback between mind and body. The degree of ease or unease in the "thinking body" results from trivial choices that may seem only marginally related to either mind or body. Tight clothes, for example, make it virtually impossible for the body to feel at ease, and thus for the mind to feel serene. The state we call "feeling fat" is actually a complex of bodymind sensations reporting a relative disparity between the size of one's body and the size of one's clothes, which is why thin people are sometimes justified in "feeling fat." I used to choose my clothes on the basis of what fit me early in the morning, which meant that whatever I wore would feel too tight—and make me feel fat—as my body expanded later in the day. Now I leave some room for expansion and feel better throughout the day as a result.

What we need is basic reeducation in simple ways of relating to our body, as summed up in the Zen recommendation "Eat when you are hungry; sleep when you are tired." A more sensible lifelong "diet plan" could scarcely be imagined.

5
Can Anxiety Make You Fat?

When we remove the tension, our body returns naturally
to its total beauty.
　　　　　　Oscar Ichazo, *Arica Psychocalisthenics*

If we boiled down all the internal obstacles to losing weight into one
word, that word would be *anxiety*. Anxiety, as both a personal trait
and a culturally conditioned response, permeates an overeater's life.
But is there a causal relationship between anxiety about your life and
getting fat? Yes. Eating more than your body wants is a compulsive
activity. It's something you wouldn't do if you were in your right
mind; you do it because you can't help yourself. J. Daniel Palm, the
author of *Diet Away Your Stress, Tension, and Anxiety,* remarks,
"Many people would gladly shed their excess pounds if they could be
free of the stress which caused them to overeat." As Chapter 6 will
discuss, some personality types (or rather, biochemical entities) are
more prone than others to engage in various forms of compulsive behavior (smoking, drinking, drug abuse, or overeating) as a means of
reducing or masking the effects of daily stress. The body is constantly
trying to keep itself in the best equilibrium possible; if you constantly
feel anxious and thereby put your body continually out of balance, it
will arrange cravings for you that will redress that imbalance. Strange
as it may sound, compulsive eating and many other addictions are the
body's way of attempting to restore health under highly adverse conditions.

Stress is a technical term, the medical name for a complex of adap-
tive bodily responses. Dr. Hans Selye, the "discoverer" of stress, warns
in *The Stress of Life* that "stress is not nervous tension." In common
usage, however, *anxiety* refers to stress translated into the language of
subjective feelings. The words *anxiety* and *stress* summon up images

of an overworked business executive ripe for a heart attack. But, as we're all coming to realize, stress affects nearly everyone in our civilization. A great deal of stress originates in the individual's habitual overreactions to problems that don't merit such a response; Palm comments, "Even [for everyday stresses] our homeostatic responses are the same as if our lives were threatened. Every time, our stress-response system mobilizes every one of the defense mechanisms which our far distant ancestors developed to keep themselves alive in their confrontations with the wild beasts."

We tend to think of stress as crisislike, a heavy sudden demand on our coping mechanisms, though it has been found that the deadliest form of stress is not sudden cataclysms (which our ancient endocrinological systems were designed to buffer, at least on an occasional basis) but chronic, low-grade, *habituated* stress—that which we are no longer conscious of. Kenneth Pelletier remarks in *Mind as Healer, Mind as Slayer* that the stresses of civilized life are ultimately more damaging than the stresses of life in the wild simply because they are so unremitting (and, he claims, cumulative in their effect): "When the source of stress is ambiguous, undefined, or prolonged, or when several sources exist simultaneously, the individual does not return to a normal mental and physiological baseline as rapidly. He or she continues to manifest a potentially damaging stress reaction."

If you are suffering from chronic stress, you may not be the only one blind to it; your doctor (likely also a chronically stress-laden individual) may not even conceive of your problem as related to stress, since the way you feel is what we define as "business as usual" in this culture. My own anecdote about being totally unconscious of gradually mounting anxiety during my Lindner Clinic experience is a good example of what I mean. For you to perceive stress as a "problem," the stressful experience would have to significantly exceed your ordinary, everyday stress threshold.

Stress may be an assault from without, but the stress response is generated internally. Dr. Selye defines the latter in *Stress without Distress* as "the nonspecific response of the body to any demand made upon it." The stress response is the body's reaction to the stressor (external event). But the *amount* of stress experienced depends uniquely on the person; as Palm says, "The stress-response changes, not the stress itself, are the bases for anxiety and tension." In his article "Stress!" Wayne Dyer writes, "If you have stress in your life, it's because *you* choose to judge people and things in a way that fills you with tension."

Our anxieties seem to us to consist of separate incidents having disparate causes—such as coping with our job, our spouse, our children, and so forth. But although we think our emotions have been elicited by outside events, this is only partly true. Habituated emotions are those that tend to perpetuate *themselves*; the "causes" are various, but the negative emotions themselves are surprisingly consistent over time. Selye writes in *The Stress of Life,* "The *internal conditioning factors* are those which have become part of the body. . . . Past experiences leave some trace, some 'tissue-memories' which influence the way we react to things."

Actually, our habituated emotions—harried thoughts and self-destructive feelings—can be seen as merely the visible results of a single misperception so indigenous to our culture that we don't see anything "abnormal" or "destructive" about it. The predominant source of stress has been defined by experts as how attached you are to having things come out the way you want. Demonstrably, anxiety is connected with our feelings about how well we are performing in our lives. We live in a culture that makes its rewards on the basis of performance; most of us are aware very early on that we are expected to perform well in order to succeed. It is as if we are constantly asking ourselves, *How am I doing? Are we doing all right? Are we doing better than the neighbors? How are the children doing? Are they doing better than the neighbors?* And so on.

Many of the artifacts of our consumer technology by their very existence set up higher and higher standards of performance. Everyone has to take higher quality pictures now that the Nikon rather than the box Brownie is the norm; everyone is expected to ski perfectly now that molded ski boots are available; everyone is supposed to turn out haute cuisine masterpieces for dinner parties instead of macaroni and cheese casseroles. And the ante is always being raised; with constant improvement in tools and equipment, all of us are forced to meet escalating standards of performance everywhere just to be considered acceptable by our peers. (Ironically, even sex, which used to afford welcome relief from performance anxiety, has now become a major *source* of it.)

Sometimes it seems utterly impossible that we could have driven ourselves onto this joyless treadmill of overachieving. Gallwey reveals,

"For most of my life I was imprisoned by the proposition that my worth as a human being could be measured by my performance. In order to be worthy of respect and love I felt that I had to perform up to certain expectations. When I succeeded, [I] would feel good; if I didn't, [I would] feel miserable." Those who carry the heaviest burden of daily, habituated stress are those who have (mistakenly) come to see all of life as a performance. Cyra McFadden's *The Serial* devastatingly satirizes a style of life in which the minutiae of everyone's habits and possessions are relentlessly scrutinized on the basis of their chic.

Since our entire culture has wholeheartedly embraced the notion of performance as a *good*, it is difficult for any of us to step back and ask Why? Why are we so fixated on performing? Why are we so enthralled with getting results? I think it's because none of us has ever been informed—or has truly believed—that we are fine *just as we are*. Our constant striving is a way of mastering inferiority feelings, of getting a little feedback that assures us we're O.K. (even though we have always had trouble believing that). The sad thing about this failure to believe in ourselves is that, as Hakuyu Taizan Maezumi points out in *The Way of Everyday Life,* "It's like a person with a pocketful of money starving to death in front of a restaurant because he's unaware of the money in his pocket."

The very notion of performing, of course, implies excelling. Compulsive people are perfectionists, who take very seriously the notion of how they are doing, and who are constantly unhappy with imperfections they perceive in their performance. As one might imagine, there is a very fine line dividing the idea of excellence from pathological perfectionism. Teenagers are the most virulent perfectionists of all, probably because, as vulnerable as they are, they understand so keenly the dire consequences of not conforming to their peers' ideas of acceptability. It is not by accident that nearly all *anorexia nervosa* victims are high-achieving teenage girls; unwittingly, they slipped over the line that separates behavior their culture applauds from an unmistakably life-endangering obsession.

Perfectionism is a marvelous way of remaining chronically dissatisfied with oneself. As a teenager, I never experienced a single moment of freedom from anxiety over my bodily self. Whenever I was fat, I was filled with self-disgust; while losing weight, I was still not happy because I couldn't be truly satisfied until I had reached my goal weight—that lowest possible number on the scale. Then, when I hit the goal weight, I effortlessly shifted gears (justifiably, as it turned out) into worrying about gaining the weight back! I claim that I've made progress along these lines since then, but sometimes I'm not so sure. One day not long ago, as I berated myself for some imperfection or other, I realized with a shock that within the last few months I had achieved several goals that had seemed utterly beyond my grasp a year earlier: I had lost thirty pounds, was no longer eating compulsively, was running one or two miles a day, and was writing this book. A year ago I would have been overjoyed even to envision these accomplishments; now that they were behind me, I took them for granted and was busy criticizing myself for some other flaw.

The trouble with being a perfectionist in an upwardly striving society is that it carries the unrealistic implications of starting out perfect and improving from there! Perfectionism means having standards that are impossible to achieve; as Theodore Isaac Rubin observes in *Forever Thin,* "As part of the obese image, there is often enormous vanity. The individual aspires to be the most beautiful person in the world. Anything less ... is seen as sheer ugliness." It also means rejecting the notion of failure. Marilyn Hassett, the actress who played Sylvia Plath in the movie version of *The Bell Jar,* commented in an interview, "One thing I learned from Sylvia is that women tend to beat themselves for anything less than perfection. But failure isn't final. It's just part of the process." Joshua Loth Liebman, the author of *Peace of Mind,* wrote:

We must cease tormenting ourselves when we do not achieve the absolute in life. We must begin to assimilate emotionally the truth that all of life is mingled failure and success, and that no man possesses a monopoly on saintliness or sin. A tolerance for the uniqueness of every human being, and a forgiveness of shortcomings—whether they be our own or those of our human comrades—these attitudes the psychological laboratories proclaim as our guarantors of serenity.

The concept of performance inevitably implies intolerance for error; our evaluation of any performance we witness (from an eight-year-old's piano recital to a dazzling solo by a professional ice skater) is always based on how few errors there were in it. But in our individual lives the rejection of failure means discrediting the best and most efficient learning tool that we possess: trial and error. I am a person who has hated making mistakes most of my life. I never wanted to be a "beginner" at anything, because my definition of adequate performance did not dip low enough to include beginners' flaws. "If I can't do it well, I won't do it at all" was my implicit thought, and therefore it was often easier for me not to do something at all rather than to struggle with it, feeling mortified at being a beginner. What idiocy!

We judge other people by objective standards—the "importance" to the world of their performance—though, curiously enough, the degree of anxiety experienced by the performer has no relation to this measure. The important government official impatiently pacing the floor or the chic society woman fussing about the arrangements for an elegant soirée may seem worlds apart from the dumpy, undistinguished grandmother worrying nonstop over some item of trivia, but their internal reactions are chemically identical. All these people are needlessly impairing their own effectiveness. I want to make clear that performing per se is not bad. All of us *must* perform. But, paradoxically, worrying about performing degrades the performance. As Dr. William Glasser explains in *Positive Addiction,* "If you are competent in anything and you can let your brain spin free while you are doing it, you will experience both more competence and more pleasure than if you keep your brain tightly controlled by conscious effort." Chronic anxiety has the same relation to accomplishment as wearing a ball and chain on your leg has to swimming.

If anything was my personal equivalent of swimming while wearing a ball and chain, it was my Ph.D. dissertation. I agonized over every word on every page, and spent more than three years writing no more than 150 pages. The present book was duck soup by comparison: I felt a great deal of anxiety about meeting the six-month publisher's deadline at first, but I recognized these feelings as merely the "learning jitters." I stayed focused and calm as much as I could, using a quieting mantra when hysteria seemed about to overwhelm me. I visualized myself writing the book speedily and willingly, even when I wasn't willing, and soon that visualization became reality: I *was* willing; I *could* write quickly. The point is, I performed two tasks of equal intrinsic difficulty; one cost me nearly ten times as much effort as the other, simply because I hadn't mastered serenity and "not-trying" and felt that worrying was a useful index of how hard I was working.

I had a personal taste of the "inner game" approach to life and performing ten years or so before Timothy Gallwey's book appeared. I was then dating the man who eventually became my second husband. He was an expert skier, and took me skiing on several weekends. Though nothing was said, I definitely felt this to be a test of my suitability as a future life companion, and therefore I felt an enormous amount of performance anxiety from the start. I had never skied before, and I felt like an uncoordinated slob. I took skiing lessons from a series of ever more intimidating instructors but seemed to only get worse instead of better. Desperate, I turned to one of our friends, an achievement-oriented skier, for a little extra help. He agreed to give me a lesson. Barking commands at me, he dragged me up and down the beginners' slope. I was nearly hysterical. I went in to lunch believing that no one, nothing whatsoever, could help me. After lunch another trusted friend, also an expert skier, said, "Come on, I'll give you a lesson." When we got off the chair lift, he said, "The first thing I want you to do is look up at the sky and drag your poles in the snow." "My God, I can't do that," I said. "I'll fall down or crash into something." "Just try it," he said. I did what he told me, and immediately began making modest but perfect little turns—entirely without assistance from my worrying conscious mind. He said, "I think you've got the idea." After a half hour or so he left me on the beginners' slope to practice, which I did until nightfall, an insanely beatific smile on my face. If I'd been a little smarter, I would have generalized his instructions to all other areas of my life immediately, rather than waiting years to see their implications.

Results are like seeds: sometimes they germinate a long time underground before flowering. This is what Emerson meant by "the long foreground"—the indirect, even invisible, preparation for a later culmination. If we think results are defined only as visible success *now,* we have missed the point. As George Leonard says in *The Ultimate Athlete,* "Numbed to everything except results, we are likely to miss the dance."

We have been made aware that this culture's "hurry sickness," or Type A behavior, is a leading predisposing stress factor in cardiac disease. According to the leading book on the subject, Meyer Friedman and Ray H. Rosenman's *Type A Behavior and Your Heart,* it is not only the Type A person's native competitiveness but also his or her "ceaseless striving, his everlasting *struggle* with time, that we believe to very frequently leads to his [or her] early demise from coronary heart disease." Dr. Richard Suinn, another expert on the Type A personality, comments in an interview that Type A people "live with time pressure as a paranoid lives with the sense that people are after him." But Type A behavior is not an isolated "problem"; it is a logical result of our culture's obsession with performance.

There should be a variant of Parkinson's Law stating that result-oriented activities expand to fill the time available. When the automobile was invented, and people could get from one activity to another faster than before, they began to engage in more of them as a matter of course. Whenever activities expand to fit the time available, however, a sense of hurry and rush is inevitable. We often talk of all the leisure-time choices our culture provides, but what we really mean is that we are being given the opportunity to feel performance anxiety about a larger number of things. We want to do all the things we define as being part of the good life, but at our backs we always hear "Time's winged chariot hurrying near." Looking for a way to squeeze everything in, we become candidates for activities as ridiculous as the "Two-Minute Yoga" that *Woman's Day* magazine offered a few years back.

Children, unfortunately, have become prime candidates for Type A overprogramming; because their talents (that is, their "results") are thought to redound to their parents' credit, they are encouraged to engage in (and, of course, excel at) as many activities as possible. In *Positive Addiction,* Glasser takes issue with this practice, arguing that unstructured time, in which the brain is allowed to "spin free," provides the best conditions for the growth of mental abilities: "I believe, therefore, that we should program our children and ourselves less completely than we do. We should allow for time off, some leeway, some slack in the day; never make it too tight."

Impatience with the God-given rate of time's passage is an insanity, but we feel the impatience anyway. When society's framework is competitive, everyone is driven by the achievement rate of the best. A book called *Stalking the Wild Pendulum* explained the concept of "rhythm entrainment," the way sensors (pendulums, living cells, etc.) synchronize themselves, usually at the rate of the fastest one in the group. The same kind of rhythm entrainment operates in human life; most of the members of a given competitive group will feel uneasy until their rate of activity matches that of the fastest achiever.

People who are focused on results want them *now.* Our natural impatience for dieting results is further inflamed by the unrealistic claims made for each new diet touted in the popular press. Each one claims weight losses of "15 pounds in nine days," or "30 or more pounds per month," neglecting to mention that to lose that much in a month a person would have to be very, very waterlogged or weigh nearly 300 pounds to begin with. If all the women's magazines in the country started a campaign to impress women that we could have our babies in less than a half-hour, without feeling a single contraction, I hope we'd have enough sense to give a horse laugh. Yet exactly the same kind of nonsensical trash about another biological process is printed month after month—and someone seems to be buying it. If believing it made it true, fine: but it doesn't. According to Barbara Brown in *Stress and the Art of Biofeedback,* "False information has been demonstrated to be inhibitory to almost all biofeedback learning." Only the truth, only reality, can help anyone find a lasting, meaningful, solution to a problem.

Anyone who accepts this culture's standards for bodily performance will experience intense frustration when his or her body does not correspond to the standards. Because overeating is a conditioned response to stress, feeling frustrated over one's weight makes one overeat in order to feel better, which intensifies the problem, ad infinitum. If one's fear of others' disapproval is great enough, it will *never* be possible to shed the anxiety long enough to learn any new behavior. (I will undoubtedly continue for the rest of my life to have impulses toward hiding empty bakery boxes deep in trash cans—behavior left over from the days when I anxiously felt I *had* to erase all traces of what I had been eating or face a highly disapproving cross-examination.)

Sadly enough, some desperate overweight people are driven to seek refuge in nonsensical solutions that contradict the basic laws of human physiology. Obese people are often ridiculed for their gullibility, for spending billions of dollars a year on shots, pills, rubber suits, slimming wafers, exercise contraptions, and every kind of unwise diet imaginable. However, this behavior is completely understandable—in fact, inevitable—in the present context. Fat people cannot reach a solution to their problem (since many steps in the instructions have always been left out), but they know that *solving the problem is mandatory*; the culture demands it. What else can be done but resort to voodoo? Victims of *anorexia nervosa* have clearly internalized the weight-fixated obsession of their culture to such a degree that they can no longer choose *not* to hold such a world view but are helpless in its grasp. Such confused people bear a strong resemblance to the laboratory rats who, after the experimenter frustrates them repeatedly beyond a certain point, begin to exhibit utterly random and irrational behavior in response to all further contact.

Recall what was said in the previous chapter about the body being an *expression* rather than a performance; that contrast needs amplification here. A performance is something we *do*; an expression is something we *are*. Ideally they are the same, though in practice they often are not. Performances need not always be "real"; in fact, we call obviously spurious performances "putting on an act." Self-expression, on the other hand, is always genuine. To allow ourselves self-expression is to be content with (or at least resigned to) ourselves as we appear to others at that moment.

Overweight people are known to be especially poor at adequate emotional self-expression, which ultimately results in their experiencing higher than normal levels of chronic anxiety. Several studies have alleged that there is an identifiable emotional-response "syndrome" characteristic of the obese personality, which includes, among other traits, passiveness, fearfulness, perfectionism, oversensitivity, the desire to please, and the wish to keep one's emotions hidden. These diverse character traits all have to do with the fact that obese people mistakenly see their personal relationships as *performances*, and they feel performance anxiety about the emotions such relationships engender. Emotions are not performances; they just *are*. There is no "right" or "wrong" about how you feel; you just feel that way. But obese people often do not give themselves permission to feel what they really feel, which has an ironically negative effect. Expressing emotions would discharge and dissipate them; suppressing them, on the other hand, turns them inward and transmutes them into stress.

Most of the books I have read about neuroses and neurotic personalities have sounded vaguely censorious, as if the reader "ought" to change him- or herself by becoming better adjusted. But this is not a realistic approach to this kind of problem. Every personality trait of every human being is not merely a series of visible actions, but a series of biochemical events as well. George Weinberg remarks in *The Action Approach,* "Whatever the person's problem, he has almost surely been told . . . that he's taking things too seriously or that he would enjoy his life more if only he'd relax. In effect, he's been told to change his adrenalin rate. . . . He's been told to exercise choice over feelings not subject to choice." The point is not that change is impossible, for it most assuredly *is* possible. But the problem is like the snake biting its tail: how do you decide where to break into the self-perpetuating vicious circle? I think the most realistic place to start is at the nutritional level, not with "will power" and self-improvement resolutions.

As Chapter 6 will explain in greater detail, a metabolic irregularity common to many types of addicts is an imbalance in the body's sugar-processing mechanism, ultimately originating in a derangement of the entire adrenocortical (stress-handling) system. The adrenalin response is what is colloquially called the fight-or-flight syndrome; it has been the body's method of dealing with stress since the beginning of time. As might be expected, the former part of the response pours out hormones to defy the attacker; the latter pours out a complementary set of hormones to ready the body to flee in fear. Biochemically, they are two sides of the same coin.

Overeaters habitually overexperience both sides of the fight-or-flight response. Anne Scott Beller reports in *Fat and Thin* that, in psychological experiments, "obese subjects were easier to frighten . . . than nonobese subjects." On the other side of the coin, Dr. Rubin compares alcoholics and overeaters in *Forever Thin:* "One of the greatest difficulties they share is an inability to handle anger. Both groups are invariably very angry people with remarkably little awareness of their anger or the ways they pervert it." Drugs and alcohol suppress the users' consciousness of things they want to forget. One of the things overeaters want to forget (repress) in order to keep their "nice guy" image intact is how angry and resentful they habitually feel at the way they are treated by the rest of society.

Overeating has a physiological rationale; it temporarily raises the sagging blood sugar of the hypoglycemic and produces a genuine—though fleeting—sense of calm and well-being. Eating is, therefore, a passport to a different and better state of mind. Raysa Rose Bonow's personal account in *How to Be a Thin Person* makes this connection startlingly explicit:

One day I was in my car, driving to a restaurant to have dinner. A terror hit me so suddenly I almost lost control of the car. I began to perspire because—I found myself thinking that I had already eaten! But how could that be? I had just left my house and was on my way to dinner. . . . My brain went rushing over the day's events. . . . All I remembered was that I was calm. CALM! I was calm. It took me a while to unravel it . . . but what I found out was so incredibly simple and so majestic in meaning for me that I am almost afraid to talk about it. . . . For a moment, my brain read CALM, and that meant I must have just eaten! WRONG! What I was feeling was the way most people feel when they are in control or are getting in control of their life and their problems.

Now, at least, we can see what the goal ought to be: to learn how to go *directly* to that desired state of mind without having to make the unnecessary detour through food. The first task is to become aware of all the messages of "un-ease" you are receiving, either from yourself or from other people or things. This will require paying close attention to your life, since, as we saw earlier in the chapter, many significant stresses will have become chronic and thus subliminal.

The second task, of course, is to eliminate as many of these as possible, or to replace them with messages of calmness and serenity, which may mean anything from adjusting tiny details such as the fit of your clothes to changing larger patterns such as your overall daily schedule. Chapter 11 provides explicit help in how to do this. One of the most important tools discussed in that chapter carries the intimidating technical name *reciprocal inhibition*—which merely means, in Barbara Brown's words, that "anxiety does not, cannot, exist when the muscles are truly relaxed." Learning how to relax your body is a precondition for learning how to relax your mind as well.

The effects of minimizing stress will be immediate and so pleasurable that they will probably continue to spread throughout your life, influencing all further choices. Dr. Selye's recommendation about choosing one's work, in his preface to Nathaniel Lande's *Mindstyles, Lifestyles,* could apply equally well to choosing a diet or an entire style of life: "Find the kind of occupation which, for us, is closest to play." It's a simply wonderful idea.

6
Messages from Your Body, 1:
The Biochemistry of Anxiety

> Nature, contrary to general opinion, does not always
> know best. Both on the cellular and interpersonal level,
> we do not always recognize what is and what is not
> worth fighting.
>
> Hans Selye, *Stress Without Distress*

The emotion we call *anxiety* is a state of body as well as of mind; if we
wished, we could think of anxiety not as an emotion but as a specific
result of nerve and hormone interaction. We are beginning to understand that events we perceive in the mind are merely the translation
into another language of the biochemical activities we call neural and
hormone processes. Indeed, this chapter is an attempt to translate the
thoughts and feelings defined as anxiety in the previous chapter into
their corresponding physiological processes. Bateson argues in *Mind
and Nature* that it is incorrect to apply logical categories such as
cause and effect to biological systems, which are characterized instead
by self-reinforcing feedback loops in which the notions of cause and
effect soon become meaningless. If in this chapter I seem to state that
hormones or blood sugar levels "cause" emotions, it is intended only as
a corrective to the prevalent view that emotions are virtually self-gen-
erating, with no basis in biology. Always I mean to imply that the process is circular, with each physiochemical event influencing a thought
or feeling that influences another physiochemical event, and so on.

J. Daniel Palm says, "Anxiety . . . is not a stress but the recognition
that a stress response has occurred." As Chapter 5 mentioned, the
stress response is a homeostatic or equilibrium-preserving (and thus
life-enhancing) process intended to keep a living creature operating
within the narrow range of variables that physiological processes admit. Recall Dr. Selye's definition of stress as "the nonspecific response
of the body to any demand made upon it." The stress response involves
the predictable sequential actions of the hypothalamus, pituitary, and

adrenal cortex and medulla. It consists of three major phases: shock, resistance, and exhaustion. The shock phase is divided into shock and countershock; the former (encounter with the stressor, which may lower blood sugar) elicits a swift outpouring of adrenalin, which brings on countershock (by raising the blood sugar and reversing many of the symptoms of shock). In countershock the hormones of the adrenal cortex are released, to carry out the work of the resistance phase. In the exhaustion phase the body's resources for fighting the stressor are finally depleted. Selye observes in *The Stress of Life,* "It is one of the most characteristic features of the [stress syndrome] that its various defensive mechanisms are always based on combinations of these two types of response: advance and retreat."

Chapter 5 mentioned that chronic stress made it progressively more difficult for the creature to respond adequately to each individual stressful event; Palm says, "When a stressful situation is prolonged or repetitious, the homeostatic mechanism of the stress response deteriorates." Isolated instances of stress begin as a response to a stimulus. But chronic stress begins to involve habituated hormonal reactions; the stress pattern has become incorporated into the body's equilibrium. As Dr. Franz Alexander writes in *Psychosomatic Medicine,* "The longer a disturbance prevails, the more complex becomes the autonomic participation. . . . In chronic conditions the neurogenic mechanisms become less important and hormonal regulations come to the foreground." Habituated hormone response in one system may then go on to derange other systems; Selye wryly observes in *The Stress of Life* that "defense may bring salvation or it may bring self-inflicted injuries." Further, chronic stress inexorably moves the creature toward exhaustion of the ability to respond to stress.

Palm remarks, "All varieties of stress, regardless of origin, result in an immediate and automatic onset of the [full-scale] stress response." Normal stress occurs in response to external events; chronic stress has become a continuously generated response to internal conditions. According to Palm, "One of the primary stresses of the body is an insufficiency of cellular fuel and of raw materials required to continue normal metabolic activities." The rest of this chapter will be devoted to examining the considerable ramifications of this single statement. A doctor friend of mine once told me, "We digest today's food with yesterday's enzymes," which means that if you spend enough yesterdays consuming manufactured food, which does not contain enough vitamins, minerals, enzymes, fiber (and perhaps even water) necessary for digestion, the body will come to lack sufficient resources to digest what you eat today. This insufficiency is a significant source of chronic stress.

Dr. John Yudkin reveals that rats fed a high sugar diet developed enlarged adrenal glands, presumably in response to the stress such a diet imposed. Dr. Robert Atkins alleges, in *Dr. Atkins' Diet Revolution,* "The more sugar you eat in your lifetime, the more abnormal your response to sugar becomes." Those who dislike admitting the deleterious effects of sugar always resort to the argument that sugar could not possibly be toxic, since glucose is the body's primary fuel. As always, it's a matter of degree; many substances that are tolerable or even beneficial in small concentrations are toxic in larger ones, and sugar and salt undeniably fall into this category.

In *Fat And Thin* Beller remarks that one notable characteristic of overweight people is that when they are given the pituitary hormone ACTH "[their] output of adrenal hormones is often two to three times greater than that of any other body type's." Overweight people may thus experience the stress response to a higher degree than others and, when they experience it too frequently, are more in danger of having it become a habituated part of their chemistry, with adverse effects upon other body functions. Dr. Melvin Page comments in *Your Body is Your Best Doctor,* "When [the endocrine] glands must meet the emergency caused by the intake of refined sugar, there is no differentiation in their influence on other functions of the body. All the cells of our body then become the unwilling victims of the overactivity or underactivity of the controlling endocrine glands."

The cells of the body that are the most vulnerable of all to the many unhealthy implications of chronic stress are brain cells. Dr. George Watson claims in *Nutrition and Your Mind* that many apparent forms of neurosis and even psychosis actually have no rational "meaning," but are merely artifacts of a derangement in the body's energy-producing mechanisms (whether too-fast or too-slow oxidation). In *Body, Mind, and Sugar* Abrahamson and Pezet comment that, of all tissues, the brain is most dependent on the moment-to-moment availability of glucose and thus most susceptible to damage if the supply is interrupted. They further allege that "a definite correlation has been established between low blood sugar, as part of a general metabolic imbalance, and certain types of insanity." E. Cheraskin et al., the authors of *Diet and Disease,* agree: "Hypoglycemia has been observed to mimic many psychiatric, somatic and neurologic disorders."

For people suffering from symptoms such as depression, despair, melancholy, and so forth, it is important to understand that such feelings may be gibberish, like a tape recording running backward. People with these feelings tend to consult solemn psychiatrists, who are willing to talk for hours about their patients' "problems"—though these may be actually nothing but the nonsensical output of a malnourished brain. When the brain receives an adequate and constant supply of glucose, neurotic symptoms can vanish—as mine did, when I learned to eat correctly.

Unfortunately many influential individuals and groups in our society have been slow to acknowledge the effects of deranged glucose metabolism upon mental functioning. Ronald M. Deutsch's *Realities of Nutrition,* disputing the existence of hypoglycemia in epidemic proportions, triumphantly stated, "There are those, however, who claim that low blood sugar afflicts a major part of our population. . . . Looking back at the claimed symptoms of hypoglycemia . . . we observe a remarkable parallel. For these are generally the symptoms of *anxiety neurosis.*" Well, of course; isn't that the point? That's what a deficiency in the body's supply of glucose from erratic blood sugar levels *does:* it intermittently starves the brain and produces the irrational symptoms of anxiety neurosis. I don't wish to quarrel with anyone over the existence of hypoglycemia; that's a semantic issue. Only the symptoms are real; they proliferate on a junk-food diet and diminish or disappear on a more sensible one. I don't need to be further convinced that alleviating the symptoms is preferable to ignoring them or masking them with antidepressant drugs.

Dr. John Tintera is quoted by William Dufty in *Sugar Blues* as saying, "It is ridiculous to talk of kinds of allergies when there is only one kind, which is adrenal glands impaired . . . by sugar." Cheraskin and Ringsdorf comment that many food allergies are compounded by hypoglycemia. Dr. Atkins adds, in *Dr. Atkins' Superenergy Diet,* "It is very difficult to make the distinction between food allergy and hypoglycemia for the simple reason that a typical food allergy involves hypoglycemia." Hypoglycemia is not a beginning of something so much as an end; it is one of the final results of a long series of equilibrium-preserving mechanisms elicited as a response to stress (when stress is chronic, hypoglycemia can become chronic, too). The initiation of the stress response is characterized by an outpouring of adrenalin, whose effect is to swiftly raise blood sugar levels to meet the purported emergency. If the adrenalin response is large and the rise in blood sugar correspondingly great, homeostatic mechanisms will come into play, eliciting insulin to bring the blood sugar level back to normal. In a deranged system both the rise in blood sugar and its consequent fall will be excessive; when the blood sugar falls to a certain (hypoglycemic) level, the stress response will be initiated in response to *that*, and the cycle simply continues.

Hypoglycemia, a frequent "shadow" to obesity, is for the slow oxidizer physiochemical type best described as *hyperinsulinism*. Too much insulin is indeed the fat person's classic double- (or even triple-) bind, since (1) it promotes the storage of fat in the body, (2) it makes it harder to burn fat already stored in the cells, and (3) it lowers blood sugar levels, increasing one's feelings of hunger. It also has a consequent adverse effect on mental functioning, as glucose levels become erratic and supply to the brain unreliable. As all anxious overeaters know, hyperinsulinism carries with it the very real threat of ultimately exhausting the pancreas and thus bringing on diabetes.

Unfortunately, people suffering from hyperinsulinism usually assuage their cravings with sugar, out of the mistaken impression that it makes them feel better. We call what they do *eating*, but it has no relation to nourishment, nor even to satisfaction. In reality it is nothing but an unceasing cycle: chronic outpouring of insulin, drop in blood sugar levels, eating of concentrated carbohydrates, rapid rise in blood sugar levels, and further outpouring of insulin, reinitiating the cycle.

Abrahamson and Pezet write in *Body, Mind, and Sugar*, "Often the question arises as to whether subclinical hyperinsulinism is the *cause* or the *effect* of accompanying illnesses. It does not make any difference." In a more stable system, each of the reactions would be less severe, keeping all the body's parameters within acceptable homeostatic limits. Keeping the blood sugar level steady can prevent this chronic stress response. Overweight people shun starchy carbohydrates (potatoes, rice, bread) like the plague, though ironically whole-grain starches—the so-called complex carbohydrates—are the best foods available for keeping blood sugar levels adequate and constant without eliciting the fat-promoting insulin response.

In *Megavitamin Therapy*, Ruth Adams and Frank Murray claim,

"Stress tends to addict us." Yes; because addictions are self-deluding attempts to escape the chronic stress-response–hypoglycemia cycle. (Dr. Atkins contends that the underlying cause of all addictions is hypoglycemia.) An addiction is a chronic allergy that has become incorporated into the body's equilibrium. Paradoxically, the outpouring of adrenalin and the rise in blood sugar at the onset of the stress response, which has been elicited by the addictive substance, *remove* the symptoms brought about by the substance's chronic toxicity. Dr. Lindner called overeating an "allergy addiction"; the body craves the high-sugar foods that give it "satisfaction" (that is, relief from hypoglycemia), though that satisfaction is temporary and illusory.

Like the stress response itself, an addiction is the body's attempt to put the creature into the least harmful equilibrium possible. All of the addictions I will consider here—alcoholism, sugar addiction, and (briefly) drug addiction—are alike in that the addictive substance acts temporarily as a stimulant but ultimately as a depressant, which requires further repeated ingestions to regain the stimulant effect. In each of these addictions the body is under stress for a variety of metabolic reasons, as we will see later. The addictive substance temporarily relieves the hypoglycemic symptoms, though it later intensifies them. On the conscious level the stress of hypoglycemia makes the addict think he or she "needs" a drink, a fix, or something sweet to eat.

William Dufty tells us in *Sugar Blues* that long ago "morphine [was used] in the treatment of sugar diabetes." It may seem surprising that what we think of as an "evil" drug was used in an effort (albeit misguided) to relieve the symptoms of a derangement of the body's sugar-processing mechanism. Morphine is a chemical cousin of the stimulants nicotine and caffeine, and like them it "mimics" adrenalin's action in the body. Morphine is very good at mimicking; in fact, its structure is so much like the body's own pain-killers (endorphins) that the body is fooled by it. Morphine "fills up" the brain's so-called opiate receptors. When the morphine fills up these receptors (thus deadening pain), a message is sent to the brain that no more endorphins are needed. As a result, when the morphine itself is finally broken down, the receptors are left empty (in pain) with no pain-killer available. The conscious mind, recalling the morphine's previous analgesic effects, thinks of using it again to stop the pain. When living cells are exposed to morphine for an extended period, they incorporate it into their metabolism, so that the morphine becomes vital to their chemistry.

In a similar fashion, caffeine and nicotine mimic adrenalin by causing a transitory rise in blood sugar, which is then lowered by insulin. Large amounts of vitamin C are consumed in the processes of both smoking and drinking coffee, as in other instances of stress. And the erratic raising and lowering of blood sugar can produce the same characteristic mental depression and fatigue. Abrahamson and Pezet state, "Caffeine is so much a causative factor in this kind of depression that the condition might be regarded as a form of caffeine poisoning."

In *Super Self* Dorothy Tennov comments that addictions are very difficult to eradicate because "acts which produce their own immediate rewards are the hardest to change. It is no accident that habits which we call 'addictive' fall into this category." Addicts continue using a drug to avoid the symptoms they know will appear if they stop using it; thus their actions are motivated by fear. In *Body, Mind, Behavior* Maggie Scarf states that "a habit motivated by fear [is] clearly, extraordinarily persistent." This is especially unfortunate since obese people tend to be significantly more fearful than others because of their higher than normal levels of epinephrine (adrenalin).

I acknowledge that the part of this chapter which treats overeating as an addiction will be very difficult for some overeaters to accept. Obese people don't mind thinking of themselves as weak-willed, despicable, or ugly; but they don't like to think of themselves as *addicts*. However, as I have argued before, trying to impose moral criteria on what is basically a physiological dilemma is wrong-headed and foolish; in fact, discussing the physiological facts behind the label may make the condition less distasteful and hence more amenable to correction. A compulsion has not only an emotional but also a biological component; in order to be rid of it, one must attack it on both levels simultaneously.

I do not insist that every reader of this book diagnose himself or herself as an addict; there are many types of overweight people and diverse etiologies of the condition. But it is clear to me that true addicted overeaters (such as I was) are the hardest of all types to cure; thus showing *them* the way to a cure may also help others with less severe problems. The "Anonymous" programs designate alcoholism, drug addiction, and overeating alike as "an allergy of the body and an obsession of the mind," though given the concept of the bodymind it might be more accurate to rephrase that as "an allergy of the body *manifested as* an obsession of the mind." First, all three diseases are disorders of chronic stress and are thus more closely related than the general public seems to understand.

The biochemical relationship between alcoholism and overeating can seem puzzling and contradictory. Stress-caused chronic hypoglycemia is common to both; in each case the addictive substance seems irresistible because it has a sedative effect on the overstressed individual (and thus puts him in a "better" equilibrium than he would be in without it). Yet at the same time the diseases are in some important ways antithetical. Lifelong alcoholics and schizophrenics are sometimes considered to have tendencies toward "personality disintegration." However, Beller has remarked that, except for their neurotic feelings about their fatness, obese people seem, on the contrary, hypernormal, hyperstable, and particularly well adjusted by all known criteria of psychological adjustment.

Alcoholics, drug addicts, and schizophrenics have in common very low levels of adrenal function, whereas obese people typically produce two to three times more adrenal hormones than normal. This particular reciprocity is the key: in terms of adrenal function, and thus reaction to stress, alcoholism and drug addiction are mirror images of compulsive overeating. To demonstrate the reciprocity, I will posit an archetypal alcoholic and an archetypal overeater representing diametrically opposite physiological types, the two ends of a continuum. (These archetypes are not, of course, people from "real life"; actual people are a mixture of characteristics somewhere along the continuum. Thus the following remarks would be overgeneralizations if applied to individuals. Further, it is possible for one person to be both an alcoholic and an overeater. But isolating the archetypal extremes can help us understand the relationship.)

Archetypal alcoholics are male ectomorphs (tall, skinny people) with high levels of thyroxin (classic examples of Watson's fast oxidizers). They may be hypoglycemic because alcohol has damaged the liver, which manufactures glycogen (sugar for storage). Their adrenal function is subnormal; that is, it does not adequately relieve the hypoglycemia. According to Beller, they lack adrenalin (epinephrine) but tend to have an excess of its counterpart, noradrenalin or norepinephrine (the hormone "related to anger"). They are not in general fearful (because they lack epinephrine, the hormone associated with fear), but disown whatever fear they do feel and therefore repress it. To a certain extent their high level of thyroxin substitutes for their deficient adrenalin. They tend to be smokers and heavy coffee drinkers because nicotine and caffeine mimic the effect of the adrenalin they lack. Their chronic hypoglycemia, which is aggravated by the fast rate at which they burn up food, is not assuaged as it is in normal people by adrenalin, because of their adrenal deficiencies; hence they select alcohol as a quick source of rapidly metabolized calories, though this paradoxically aggravates their basic metabolic problem. The alcohol produces a sedative effect when first ingested, though the effect is short-lived. According to Null and Null's *Alcohol and Nutrition,* "All recovered alcoholics [in a given test group] were hypoglycemic. This tended to be chronic and was apparently the result of a dysfunction in the [adrenocortical] system." Null and Null further observe that the symptoms of delirium tremens are similar to those of Addison's disease, a malady of adrenocortical insufficiency.

Archetypal overeaters represent the obverse of most of these traits. Typically female endomorphs (rounded, fleshy people), they tend to be subnormal in thyroxin (therefore, in Watson's terminology, slow oxidizers). Because of their high levels of adrenalin output, fear is the dominant neurotic expression of their personalities; whatever anger they feel, they tend to disown and repress. As slow oxidizers, they tend to have high blood glucose levels. When they are under stress, large secretions of adrenalin further raise their glucose levels, which in turn calls forth an excessive insulin response, which both mediates the storage of glucose as fat and lowers blood glucose again to the level at which the stress response is initiated. Their hypoglycemia, unlike that of the alcoholic, is more correctly termed hyperinsulinism. For overeaters sedation is achieved both by the transitory raising of the blood sugar levels through concentrated carbohydrate intake and by what Beller describes as the "sedative effect that insulin produces as it goes about moving sugar into the cells and simultaneously removing glucose from the blood."

In *The Stress of Life* Dr. Selye observes that "many of the so-called metabolic diseases are also largely diseases of adaptation," in other words, involving the stress response. Several component parts of the stress response themselves predispose the person to further fat formation. The first of these is the way that the stress response encourages sodium retention in the body. Dr. Yudkin reports an experiment in which rats with their adrenal glands removed preferred salt water to pure water, apparently because the salt mimicked the sodium-elevating effect of the missing adrenal hormones. The normal balance between sodium and potassium outside the cells (in the serum) is disturbed by the onset of the stress response; two of the adrenal cortical hormones, aldosterone and cortisol, act to retain sodium and excrete potassium. This can be unhealthy; as Adelle Davis remarks in *Let's Eat Right to Keep Fit,* "If stress causes the production of one's [adrenal hormones] to be far above normal, so much sodium is held in the body that a severe and dangerous potassium deficiency can occur." The water will be excreted only when the blood sugar level remains stable above that which initiated the stress response. Thus chronic stress can be the cause of chronic water retention, which will cease only when the stress itself ceases. Unfortunately, high sodium levels by themselves make it easier to get fat; according to Beller, "High sodium counts at the cell walls seem to markedly improve the cell's ability to take up glucose." The implications of excessive body sodium in hypertension (another condition that frequently "shadows" obesity) are already well known.

The second factor predisposing to obesity is excess insulin, for all the reasons discussed earlier in the chapter. Whereas water retention is a relatively simple problem to solve merely by avoiding stress and changing to a diet much lower in sodium, the problem of excess insulin is more complex, particularly for women. Insulin output in the female seems to vary with age. As Beller explains it, because pregnant women need to regulate not only their own blood sugar but also that of the fetus, their insulin mechanism may become damaged during pregnancy, apparently as a result of exposure to high levels of estrogen (this is why pregnancy is often called a diabetes-causing disease). Another precursor of maturity-onset diabetes (occurring even in women who have never borne children) is increasing insensitivity of the cells to insulin, requiring the body to continue producing it in ever larger quantities—which may ultimately exhaust the pancreas and lead to diabetes. Menopause removes the last obstacle to unrestricted fat formation in the female by shutting off estrogen, an important insulin antagonist. Beller says, "Middle-aged spread is an estrogen deficiency disease of women with faulty insulin balance." Even without these physiological predispositions, however, an unwise diet can in and of itself unbalance insulin production.

Obese people tend to see themselves as unfortunate victims of their metabolism, though that view evades a fundamental question of responsibility. In *Mind as Healer, Mind as Slayer* Pelletier remarks that "when a prolonged neurophysiological stress response is channeled through a particular personality configuration, a specific disorder will result." Life continually offers the opportunity for choices. The chronic stress–hyperinsulinism–sugar addiction syndrome *can* be reversed if one takes care to minimize stress wherever it occurs in one's life. In *The Stress of Life* Selye makes quite clear the relationship between dietary choices and the amount of stress an individual experiences. He mentions diet as an example of the "internal conditioning factors" which "have become part of the body," and then states, "Take the case of conditioning by food substances. The same amount of proinflammatory (mineralocorticoid) hormone which causes marked kidney damage and hypertension in a rat kept on a high salt intake has absolutely no such effect if given to a rat receiving a salt-free diet." R. O. Brennan and W. C. Mulligan, the authors of *Nutrigenetics,* say, "Functional hypoglycemia is caused when an individual who suffers from a specific genetic weakness fails to strengthen it with nutritious eating. The cause then is *nutrigenetic*, a combined form of nutritive and genetic influence."

This chapter may sound like the standard what-a-problem-we-have-here treatise found in most books on obesity. But that isn't the whole story. Our culture's objections to obesity on grounds of health and aesthetics have produced a certain myopia in which obese people are seen in terms of *only* their present problems, not their undeniable strengths and future possibilities. Beller points out that the ability to store fat was once a survival-promoting characteristic, though the same condition is now considered a disease.

But Dr. J. A. Winter, in *Why We Get Sick*, defines disease as a "mistaken path toward health." Obesity is probably the clearest example of the truth of that statement. We can logically assume that those who possess some (formerly) survival-promoting traits are the winners of the evolutionary race. Though the tendency to secrete large amounts of insulin today seems like a vulnerability rather than an advantage, even now we can see vestiges of its former utility. (Melvin

Page observes, "One of the most important functions of insulin is fighting infection.") High levels of adrenalin, now counterproductive in an age of constant, relentless stress, was once the most valuable trump card of all, the creature's assurance of triumphing against severe adversities.

The earlier part of this chapter demonstrated that many of the separate issues making up the "problem" called obesity (mental derangement, fatigue, fat formation, water retention, and hypertension, among others) can be separate manifestations of *one problem*: endocrine overresponse to stress. Isn't it obvious that this is cause not for alarm but for rejoicing? Except for the results of their overreactive adrenals (which can be mitigated by sensible life choices), overweight people are models of optimum functioning. Some of the words Beller uses as she describes the results of various studies comparing obese populations with normal people are *more sexually appetitive, perseverative, single-minded, significantly brighter, better information processors, having great sensory susceptibility and receptivity,* and *able to produce order out of chaos.* She remarks, "The image that begins to emerge from these new data is that of an affective powerhouse, slow to rouse initially but intensely reactive once aroused; emotionally susceptible and vulnerable, and capable of more than ordinary emotional intensity once moved; single-minded and hard to distract under ordinary circumstances, but highly distractible when the stimulus is emotionally unpleasant or otherwise negatively charged."

The poor self-image of obese people is a gift from their culture, their excessive fearfulness the inevitable result of an oversupply of epinephrine, and the sickliness and ungainliness of an obese body a foregone conclusion. But these "problems" can spring from a single basic cause and thus are amenable to a single basic solution. Here we're talking about a fairly simple and inexpensive method by means of which an obese person can *solve* the problem for good, which means *never having to think about it again.* I know that this is possible, for I am a living example of it, and if *I* can do it, *anyone* can.

I hope this chapter has provided convincing evidence that for overweight people stress is lethal. Eliminating all possible sources of it in one's body and mind is the best and surest way to return one's body to normal, joyful—and *thin*—operation. I think it's at least worth a try.

7
Resistance versus Growth

The river delights to lift us free, if only we dare let go.
Richard Bach, *Illusions*

The balance between growing (that is, changing) and staying the same is central to all living individuals and systems. Each discipline has its own name for the phenomenon (in politics, for example, it is called liberal versus conservative, or progressive versus reactionary). As earlier chapters have explained, physiological equilibrium, or homeostasis, is the center point toward which the body's daily fluctuations are always returning. This is the major mechanism by which any living creature remains who he is in the face of constant cellular change; if there existed no pattern or idea for bodily processes to return to, change would be random, unpredictable, cancerous. Such a balance also characterizes the universe as a whole; as Suzuki expresses it in *Zen Mind, Beginner's Mind,* "Whatever we see is changing, losing its balance. The reason everything looks beautiful is because it is out of balance, but its background is always in perfect harmony. This is how everything exists ... losing its balance against a background of perfect balance."

But growth—the irresistible life principle—is what makes the body's equilibrium truly a dynamic, not static, condition, a series of exquisitely poised fluctuations and rhythms. We don't have to choose growth; as living systems we are compelled to it. "Growth" means not only the simple, ceaseless process of cell replacement, but also the permanent changes in the individual that occur as a result of learning from life experiences. The imperatives of growth are seen most clearly in children, who seem propelled along some inner path, adding new abilities and characteristics at each turn. Adults, on the other hand, can choose to slow the pace of change or growth nearly to a standstill by defining themselves in given (self-limiting) ways, then believing that definition. Soon all perceptions form themselves around this controlling idea, and other possibilities begin to atrophy. Mildred Newman and Bernard Berkowitz, in *How to Be Your Own Best Friend*, counsel a more flexible approach: "When you insist you're not the kind of person who can climb a mountain or make a speech, all you are saying is that up to now you haven't done it. . . . That's what growth is."

You are reading this book because you think you want to be different—very different—from what you are now, and you may be a trifle peeved to have me waste your time by dwelling on how potent the forces are that keep each of us the same throughout our lives. The issue is important only because I hope to persuade you not to set up unreal expectations or deadlines that your body will be unable to fulfill. This chapter is a pivot point in the book. The chapters before it have been concerned with the problem; those after it deal with solutions. This chapter is meant to be a long, hard look at the arguments on both sides: the rewards of staying the same versus those of changing. I believe that many people fail repeatedly in their efforts to lose weight only because they have never fully acknowledged the part of them that resists change and wants things to stay the way they have always been. As Timothy Gallwey says: "That part of you which wants to strengthen its will to win is *only* a part. There are other elements in your makeup which are content with the way things are, and still others which will resist any kind of increase in your determination. This is perfectly natural."

It is true that in the rest of this chapter resistance is often defined as the villain, that negative part of us that keeps us from getting where we want to go. But before getting carried away with moral strictures, let us remember that resistance is defined much less prejudicially in other fields of endeavor. Resistance in an electric current, for example, is the force that impedes the electrons' progress through the wire. It's customarily expressed simply as R, an integral part of the conductivity equation—a given, one facet of how reality works. In *Steps to an Ecology of Mind* Bateson defines cybernetic reality as incorporating resistance, or restraints: "In cybernetic language, the course of events is said to be subject to *restraints,* [without which] the pathways of change would be governed only by equality of probability."

There is a definite difference between simple stasis and resistance. I use *stasis* to denote staying-the-same as a proper response (like a possum's "freezing" to fool a predator). *Resistance* is the word used when learning needs to to be done, when change would be appropriate but the organism can't or won't make the proper response. The refusal to change is a condition of willed inertia; as W. H. Auden gloomily saw it, "We would rather be ruined than changed." According to Dr. Martin Schiff in his weight loss guide, "Many people don't want to lose their problem. Their mind has dwelt on it continuously for such a long time that it is almost the same as losing a close friend." The psychiatrist Roger Gould once gave a more sympathetic account in an interview of why we find change so threatening: "Change is interpreted by us as an abandonment process—we are leaving who we were and leaving the people who knew and accepted us that way. And our delicate, complicated relationships with close people are disturbed when we change. They know us in a certain sort of way and have a stake in our not changing. We're a part of their security pattern."

There are only two types of barriers to progress in any self-improvement endeavor. The first is simple ignorance—not understanding what mechanisms lead to the solution. For several centuries our civilization has been highly successful in relentlessly diminishing our collective ignorance about the facts and mechanisms of the natural world. Consider all the diseases our ancestors used to die from because no cure could exist until the etiology of the disease was understood. Today a person could still contract the same diseases, but in our culture dying from them would be a perverse choice, not an inevitable fact. Without ignorance, the solution to any problem would be straightforward except for internal resistances, that is, attitudes that keep us from solving a given problem even though we already possess all the necessary information. As my friends the marriage counselors Jordan and Margie Paul once said, "The question is never 'how to' but 'why not'?" In fact, not just this chapter but the entire book is resistance-oriented, since I believe that (1) in the field of weight control all the "how-to's" have been appropriately identified, and (2) once you find out what resistances are keeping you from doing these, your problem will solve itself without further agonies of "will power" or titanic struggles for self-control.

Before your resistances will go away, it's very important to ask whether they have any value to you at all. Susan Newton once observed, "Either overweight serves some positive function in your life, or you're afraid of being thin for some reason." Once acknowledged, a resistance could become a vital part of your self-awareness: identifying what you felt might eventually allow you to choose to feel another way instead. Fritz Perls likened resistance to tensing a muscle; once you can *feel* that it's tense, you can learn how to relax it.

Unfortunately, dieters' resistances often show up as excuses, rationalizations, or even outright lies used to explain away excess poundage or out-of-control behavior. Of course, our excuses, transparent and pitiful as they are, will always seem silly to others; but that does not alter the fact that the reasons behind them either are now or once were valid. It is extremely important that you not accept your critics' point of view and adopt a harsh, judgmental attitude toward yourself as you look at all the minor dishonesties that compose your personal collection of resistances about overeating. If you are deeply ashamed of something about yourself, your inner being will simply repress it rather than permit you to examine it honestly and thoroughly. (Remember that the principal charter of the bodymind is to keep you as stress-free as possible; unfortunately, self-deceit is often necessary to accomplish this goal.)

Your resistances to solving your problem are much greater, and run much deeper, than you know. In fact, taken together, your resistances form a perceptual bias that helps determine your present bodymind equilibrium. This is expressed more colloquially, but no less clearly, in Castaneda's *The Second Ring of Power:* " 'The Nagual said that all of us throughout our lives develop one direction to look,' she went on. 'That becomes the direction of the eyes of the spirit. Through the years that direction becomes overused, and weak and unpleasant, and since we are bound to that particular direction we become weak and unpleasant ourselves.' "

The most prevalent type of self-deceit concerning overeating and overweight is failing to acknowledge how complex the problem is and how many factors must work harmoniously (and simultaneously) for it to be solved. Dieters persist in chasing after the illusions of Eternal Thinness via two weeks' worth of monotonous food, averting their eyes from physiological realities over and over again. Your resistance to allowing your bodymind to make choices that would eventually cause you to be thin is all tied up with your wanting things to remain familiar. As Laurence Reich explained in *From Fat to Skinny*, "Whatever the change, we are usually unprepared for it. We cannot foresee the outcome, and so most of us find it threatening. That is, until after the change has been accomplished. Before and during the process, we tend to see change from a negative point of view." The point is, you don't *need* to have things the way they have always been; you merely *want* them that way. Remember the comparison in Chapter 3 of dieting with visiting an unfamiliar foreign country: when you feel disoriented and uncomfortable, you are encouraged to give up without accomplishing anything. Learning always involves some alteration of the previous mental paradigm; resistance can thus be defined as the feeling of discomfort you experience before the new paradigm becomes perfectly clear.

Not only do resistances serve the function of protecting the ego structure, often they *are* the ego structure (and thus, naturally, they operate subliminally). We often talk about various defense mechanisms in the personality, but it would be more accurate to say that the entire personality is a defense mechanism. My husband and I once spent some months in a personal-growth discussion group for couples. As we all got to know each other better, an amusing thing happened. Each one of us was the "target" of the group at some point or other; without exception, each of us heatedly denied possessing whatever disagreeable trait the other group members could clearly see was the biggest source of trouble in our lives. I once heard Harvey Jackins, the founder of Re-evaluation Counseling Therapy, explain in a lecture that our brains are like tape recorders inside our heads. Every so often a few feet of tape are snarled and jammed and won't play properly; these small snarls we call our "problems." But right in the middle a huge segment of the tape is all jammed up, impossible to either decipher or untangle—and this we call our "personality."

To put it bluntly, you say with your mouth that you want to be thin, but all your actions and thoughts are those of a fat person. You subliminally identify with your resistances, claiming that they are "you." When you read diet books that tell you to enjoy lettuce and cottage cheese more, or spend at least a half-hour a day exercising, you inwardly bridle at the thought. Probably no one has ever pointed out to you that all of your personal preferences are nothing more than arbitrary choices; they could just as easily be something else. As Don Juan tells Carlos in *Journey to Ixtlan,* "People hardly ever realize that we can cut anything from our lives, any time, just like that."

In Western culture we have always been so infatuated with the natterings of our conscious minds (which we fatuously call our "ideas") that we cannot see them for what they really are—arbitrary constructs. To Buddhists conscious thoughts are merely the repetitive turning of the mind's squirrel cage. Your fat thoughts are not reality; they are merely the arbitrarily placed furnishings of your conscious mind. What you need to accomplish is a mental interior redecoration. Marcel Proust wrote in *Remembrance of Things Past,* "A man cannot change, that is to say become another person, while he continues to obey the dictates of the self he has ceased to be." Elsewhere in this book I have talked about trial and error as the best possible learning method; think of resistance as the best and most unfailing way to get stuck in the error part.

Which of all your thoughts about yourself are the ones that keep you from changing? They are whatever you find immensely painful to admit about yourself, whatever you think you should keep hidden out of fear that others won't like you. This part of you is called your "disowned self"—the part of you you're too ashamed to acknowledge. As I said earlier, things about yourself that you're ashamed of are things you will simply not be able to bring yourself to examine clearly for the purpose of gaining awareness. Overweight people are known to be especially good at hiding things—not just bakery boxes, but feelings as well. Resistance is an inevitable response if you feel constantly criticized or belittled by friends and family. Wanting to be thought of as "nice," fat people hide and repress their rage at a world that devalues them and constantly nags at them to be different from what they are. Resentment is hidden anger, bottled up instead of being expressed and thus discharged. It is poison to compulsive people. In addition, keeping your self-esteem precariously protected by hiding your behavior and your feelings locks you into a profound and irretrievable loneliness. I spent many years there; looking back, it's quite clear that the price I had to pay in candor about my condition was well worth being released from the burden of my self-consciousness.

Let's say you've read the description of resistance and have definitely decided to opt for growth. You decide to set your mind a little harder to what you're doing, use a little more will power, and hope for the best this time. It won't work. As I said earlier, your resistances run much deeper than you know; in fact, they are an integral part of your present state of equilibrium. A deficiency of will power is not the problem, and it cannot be cured by more "self-control." Self-control is identical to "trying"; it implies anxiety about the success of the outcome. When you decide to control yourself more, you may *seem* to be choosing change, but you're not: you're still stuck in all your old ways of thinking. "We don't *think* about it," Ira Progoff once said about his Intensive Journal process in an interview. "For if we did, we would only have the same thoughts we have always had. We know from experience that self-analytic, self-judgmental thinking tends to move in circular grooves, repeating itself. We wish instead to open the way for something new to enter our experience."

Right here is the crux of the entire book: the people who most need to understand that will power and "trying" are not the ways to solve the problem are by definition those constitutionally incapable of perceiving that fact. Compulsive, anxiety-ridden people (with their peculiar biochemical constitution that reinstates these thoughts and feelings constantly) are people who firmly believe that effort, trying, and worrying are the only ways to get what they want. If they didn't think that way, they wouldn't be the people they are, and they wouldn't have the problem in the first place. The number who change are few indeed. One of my friends, a confirmed Type A person, complained to me about the meditative exercises I had suggested to help her get rid of her chronic anxieties. "Nancy," she said, "I just can't sit still and be quiet like you're supposed to be when you do those." That's the entire problem, right there. As Don Juan says in Castaneda's *The Second Ring of Power,* "[People] love to be told what to do, but they love even more to fight and not do what they are told."

If going around in habituated circles felt completely comfortable, no impetus would exist for significant change. Fat people don't usually feel comfortable, though; they feel miserable. Overweight people are thought to have a very low tolerance for emotional discomfort; in fact, compulsive eating is usually seen as an attempt to escape such pain. Actually, there are two kinds of pain: one guarantees that you will stay the same, and the other changes you. The former is a powerful agent of resistance, the latter of growth. The former could more properly be called self-punishment; it is the state of mind in which you insist on hanging onto all your self-deprecating ideas. It is being stuck: insisting on your "wants," your "pride," your ability to blame someone or something else for your problem, or your fear of the unfamiliar. You are guaranteed to keep on experiencing all the pain associated with staying fat if you refuse to see that what is required is a fundamentally new approach to the problem.

In *Design for a Brain,* W. Ross Ashby comments, "How defenceless is the organism when pain has not its usual effect of causing be-haviour to change." At some point in every former fat person's life there came a time at which the pain of being fat was so intense and all-encompassing that it jolted that person right out of all those self-defeating circular thoughts and dishonest, repetitive behavior. To "get it" means basically to become so uncomfortable that you're forced into new ways of thinking. A standard catch phrase of Alcoholics Anonymous is "It takes what it takes," which simply means that each person has a predetermined level of frustration over his or her out-of-control behavior which will finally let him or her drop the defenses and seek help. Each person must experience this level of pain before any meaningful change can occur. Change never comes easy; that's why, as Joseph Chilton Pearce points out, "In mythology every Tree of Life is guarded by a dragon, a monster hideous and deadly to behold."

Once the arbitrariness of your resistances and the shortcomings of your attempts at "trying" become apparent to you, then you are open to learning, ready to entertain the crucial distinction between What I Want and What I Need. I remember once hotly debating this distinc-tion in a group; at the time none of us got the point. We thought it was nothing more than semantic hairsplitting. It isn't, though. What I Want is to behave according to the dictates of my resistances; What I Need is to learn behavior that brings me back to wholeness and health, often by a route opposite to What I Want. For example, for someone who had been a solitary person all his life and found himself ill at ease in groups, What I Want would be to be left alone; What I Need would be to gradually learn how to feel more self-assured around people. The growth process would seem uncomfortable at first; as Richard Corriere and Joseph Hart put it in The Dream Makers, "Everybody wants something special, but few want to go through what they must to attain it." But there is the payoff. "We either make our-selves miserable, or we make ourselves strong. The amount of work is the same," as Don Juan observed in Castaneda's Tales of Power.

Earlier in the chapter I said that resistances often manifested them-selves as excuses. However, excuses and rationalizations and lies are only the visible part of your collection of resistances. The largest part of the collection is invisible, because it consists of habituated messages you have been continually sending yourself. You have chosen not to bring them to conscious awareness before because you were ashamed of them and felt better not having to face them. You must become aware of them, however, before you can hope to get rid of them, which means you have to be willing to look.

Perhaps the largest new source of pain as you journey toward self-discovery will be the uncomfortable feelings connected with being honest with yourself for the first time—honest about how much you eat, about your negative emotions, about practically anything. I still remember vividly how ashamed I always felt when forced to admit anything about my eating (as in guiltily answering a family member who asked, "Who ate all the rest of the cookies?"). I am not a preacher; my recommendation of unequivocal self-honesty has no moral basis. For me the only issue is cybernetic. Dishonesty is not *bad*, but it does impair the quality of feedback, and correct feedback is everything. Go without it and you will cripple your attempts to change your old being into something better.

After you become aware of a certain obstacle to growth (for example, my becoming aware that the kitchen was full of cues for me to start eating), you then have to decide to take action (I have to decide if I'm willing to stay out of the kitchen or not). The willingness to take action is crucial. J.A. Winter says that whenever people say, "I wish" (as in "I wish I could be thin"), what they really mean is "I think I want this, but I'm not going to take any action." This is basically an undisciplined approach to getting what we want.

What's wrong is our interpretation of the term *discipline*. We think of it as synonymous with *deprivation,* in other words, something that makes us unhappy. But as Colette once said to a whiner, "Who said you should be happy? Do your work." She also observed, "I already know that discipline is the cure for every ill." Our Puritan heritage is at fault for indoctrinating us with the tyrannical notion of "should," an unduly harsh view of what discipline means. Besides being unnecessarily punitive, this approach simply contradicts all the known facts about how to effectively deliver one's instructions to the bodymind. Susan Newton once told me, "Never say to yourself that you *should* do something. Your unconscious mind interprets that as 'I don't want to.'" Obviously, you would never say "should" in reference to something you were just yearning to do, only something you found unappetizing. Effort is required to reach the goal, but not clenched teeth.

The *Twelve Steps and Twelve Traditions* of Alcoholics Anonymous describes the passage into disciplined behavior as "like the opening of a door which to all appearances is still closed and locked. All we need is a key, and the decision to swing the door open. There is only one key, and it is called willingness. Once unlocked by willingness, the door opens almost of itself."

This, then, is the true meaning of growth: changing and learning, but within the structure of a discipline. According to the "Big Book" of Alcoholics Anonymous, "The only real freedom a human being can ever know is doing what you ought to do because you want to do it." The steps you take within the confines of the discipline can be as small as necessary; no one needs to make progress according to some fixed scheme. In an article called "The New Discipline" Amy Gross wrote an eloquent, moving paean to the joys of discipline:

With discipline, one has a handle on life. Without it, one is constantly burning one's hand on the pot. With discipline, one comes as close to having a fairy godmother as real life allows. One has a technique for reaching from wish to fulfillment. Without discipline, one can only stare like a window-shopper at the good things in life, and shrug, and move on. . . . Discipline is one of the thirty or so names for the secret of living.

I must admit that of all the chapters in the book, this one is dearest to my heart. On the surface it may seem an objective discussion of the issues, but underneath it is my personal story. I was born resistant; each stage of my growth was accompanied by great emotional upheavals. I could never just accept things as they were; I had to agonize over everything. School counselors noticed it and told me; my parents told me; boyfriends told me. I always heard, "Gee, you take things so *hard,*" or "Try and take it easy." One therapy group meeting I attended a few years ago featured a meditative exercise in which we were to listen for a word that would be spoken from deep within, a kind of mystical slogan expressing our inmost self. As I listened attentively, the phrase that came up from my depths was "I *won't.*"

Remember what I said earlier in the chapter about having all the facts yet being unable to take the action that would solve the problem? That's me. As might be expected, I always instinctively trusted my mind but basically distrusted (or rather despised) my body. I never paid any attention to body signals. I always phrased my goals negatively; my wish to change always originated in self-disgust. I had a lot of "remedial" work to do just to become minimally aware of what was really going on in my bodymind, then become willing to trust that part of me.

I once had all the classic food resistances. Several books have enumerated the standard ones; all I have to add is that I never heard anyone else's excuses without feeling they were my own.

- There's not enough of that to put back in the refrigerator; I'll finish it.
- I was only going to have *one,* but they were so good!
- The kids really like these; I'd better buy some more.
- I think I'll stock up for the weekend in case someone comes over.
- I'm feeling kind of weak; I'd better go get a doughnut (candy bar, cookies).
- I can't start dieting now—it's Friday.
- I'll start my diet again *next* Monday.
- I felt cooped up all day; let's go out for dinner.
- Don't you want that dessert? Can I have it, then?

For years I could never get a workable, steady exercise program started; every time I would think about exercises, my resistances would come out in full force:

- Who will look after the children while I'm doing this?
- I just don't have enough time for it.
- That hill is too steep for me.
- That asphalt is too hard to run on.
- I'll never find a parking place close to the track.
- I don't want all those other people looking at me in my shorts.
- I look so lumpy in sweatpants.
- I just can't get to work on time if I run beforehand.
- It's raining (too hot, too cold, too dry).
- My ankles (knees, calf muscles) hurt.
- My life is too unpredictable for me to commit myself to this.

Throughout my life, however, anomalies in both my eating and exercising had occurred, always during the high-energy periods of spontaneous weight loss. Now I know that the mechanism behind this sudden and puzzling shift in the activities I claimed I "liked to do" was merely that I sustained a more flattering image of myself, and that for this idea to be expressed in reality, my behavior and preferences simply had to change—and they did, spontaneously.

I can laugh now about the silliness of all my former resistances, just as I can laugh (a bit ruefully) about the silly things I did when I was an immature high school sophomore. The point is that I no longer have to act out any of them. My sense of being pleasingly connected with reality is contingent upon my sustaining disciplined behavior. Willingness is the only key.

If you can't feel willing right now, don't automatically flagellate yourself. Everyone's progress away from resistance happens at an individual rate. You may even have to read this chapter many times before your problem disappears for good, and there's nothing wrong with that. I will always cherish David A. Schoenstadt's *The San Francisco Weight-Loss Method* because of the way it sympathetically urges the reader not to despair because of a failure or two:

If you didn't succeed this time, do me this favor. Don't rush out for another diet book a friend just told you about. You've bought the last fat book you'll ever need. It's honest, it's workable, it's safe, and when you are ready to succeed, it will tell you how. Put this book on the shelf. Wait awhile and try again. I failed four times on the stationary bicycle before I finally got back on and rode into this new world.

Keep asking yourself, "What *am* I willing to do?" and then do that. And keep in your head one memorable resolution from *Twelve Steps and Twelve Traditions* of Alcoholics Anonymous: "This I cannot do today, perhaps, but I can stop crying out 'No, never.' "

THE SOLUTION

8

The Illusion of Control

The true purpose is to see things as they are, to observe
things as they are, and to let everything go as it goes.
This is to put everything under control in the widest
sense.

Shunryu Suzuki, *Zen Mind, Beginner's Mind*

The belief that we can and should control ourselves by the exercise of
the conscious will is one of the most deep-seated and pervasive illusions in all of Western culture. I cannot hope to dispel it in this brief
chapter, but I can take issue with some of its basic assumptions and
sketch an alternative system that is much more effective for solving
personal problems. As I've said before, if what we were already doing
was working, we'd have no need for discussions like this one. But it
isn't working; our problems *aren't* getting solved. We need an entirely
new mental perspective in order to discover how to proceed.

Our entire culture is a society of "doing" rather than "being." The
whole show runs on a narrow set of principles: try and try again, do
and do some more, achieve, achieve, achieve. All of us believe that
anything we have of value—possessions, jobs, status, awards, relationships—came about because of our striving to get them. I used to believe this implicitly; in fact, the only thing I knew how to do was "do";
it was the only thing I ever thought necessary to learn, or anyone saw
fit to teach me. Learning "not-doing" was as hard as anything I've
ever tried to grasp. (Notice that when you talk about "not-doing," all
the words available to describe it sound like still more doing.)

This chapter's viewpoint is that an individual's errors in how to
think are nothing more than the culture's biases writ small. We have
every reason to think the thoughts our culture teaches us to think,
even if they're wrong; but if we're not happy with the results, we also
have the right to examine reality for ourselves and then change our

minds to provide a better fit between our ideas and the way things really are.

Chapter 5 tried to make clear that the amount of stress we experience is directly connected to how attached we are to having things come out the way we want. Clearly our attachment to results is linked to a strong desire to *control* events—to manipulate until everything comes out as we want it to. All of us are mixtures of control-your-life versus accept-what-you've-got traits, but it's safe to say that compulsive people are very highly developed in the control sphere and correspondingly atrophied in their ability to accept.

A passive attitude is foreign to us, since we have become highly accustomed to and comfortable with "doing"; we equate passiveness with laziness or inanition, thinking that it can't help us reach our goals. It is important to note, however, that giving up control by the conscious will is not the same as opting for aimlessness. At an Inner Skiing workshop I once attended we were shown an exercise whose idea was to keep our bodies *neither* limp *nor* rigid; we were simply to be alert and focused upon our intent. Aimlessness is the equivalent of "limp"; nothing is accomplished. Rigidity paralyzes us in the attempt to get to the goal. Relaxed, focused, nonself-conscious effort is the most efficient path to success.

Those who believe most strongly that "will power" and "self-control" are the necessary tools for subduing one's rampant desires are also those most resentful of attempts at control imposed from without. (These are the people who buy diet books in great numbers, but who—as I did—mentally resist any specific weight loss suggestions.) Priding themselves as they do on their ability to control contingencies, compulsive people are keenly embarrassed by themselves whenever they exhibit out-of-control behavior—which is why so many compulsive people have trouble admitting their compulsions.

Since most of us believe in the virtue of—not to mention the imperative of—self-control, we find it a strange and threatening idea to relinquish such control in favor of "letting go." The implicit question for dieters is always, "If I give up trying, won't I just simply balloon up to 300 pounds?" Faced with these fears about the dire consequences of freedom, most people cannot bring themselves to "give up." Dr. Lindner once told me that—statistically—modestly overweight people have a much smaller chance of solving their weight problem than grossly obese people. The reason seems to be that for the former "will power" or "controlling themselves" had always seemed to work, at least to a point. Deviating from the rigid methods they had always used in order to learn a new, more successful method from someone else was a terrifying threat to them; they thought giving up controlling themselves in their old ways would immediately turn them into enormous blimps. Severely obese people could be more easily persuaded to give up their own strategies in favor of someone else's method since their own attempts had obviously not worked. Closer to despair, they were also closer to that state of receptive humility that made it possible to genuinely accept and use the help that was offered from outside.

Compulsive eating is, among other things, Type A behavior expressed by means of food. We are Type A dieters, too. The hardest thing for any control-oriented dieter to give up is anxiety over when the diet will be over with. Even after I had come to terms with what foods I would eat, what times to eat, and so forth, I still found myself thinking, "When will I ever be *through* with this?" A natural question, granted; but if the question is repeated to the point that it creates mental unease, then it is clearly counterproductive.

The attitude is especially counterproductive when it is coupled with expectations that are biologically naive, to say the least. We have become so insensitive to our body's own tempo that we try to run it as if it were a corporation—by means of directives issued from above. If you have acquired your ideas about how fast you "should" lose weight from current conventional wisdom, you may feel highly critical of your actual performance, though only your actual performance, not the magazine article you read, represents reality. I have never read a diet article that didn't counsel patience about the rate of weight loss, but what the authors didn't seem to understand was that anyone who needed to read that article had the problem they had *because* of their inability to apply patience and serenity to the task at hand.

While I personally identify with the impatience of all compulsive people, I am also struck by the silliness of it; after all, life is not an enterprise in which one gets extra points for finishing early. Losing weight is fundamentally a learning process. If we were in college, majoring in chemistry, let's say, we wouldn't assume that one twelve-week course would immediately give us all the knowledge we needed for professional success. We do feel that way about losing weight, however; twelve weeks seems an incredibly long time to anyone on a diet.

But all the moral strictures in the world about how we "shouldn't" want to control things are only half as effective as the simple demonstration that control is a strategy that *does not work*. We are pragmatists, and the does-it-work argument is one we listen to attentively. Chögyma Trungpa's argument in *Cutting Through Spiritual Materialism* is, "You do not constantly have to manage yourself. You must disown rather than attempt to maintain control, trust yourself rather than check yourself. The more you try to check yourself, the greater the possibility of interrupting the natural play and growth of the situation." In *The Medusa and the Snail,* Dr. Lewis Thomas explains why this is so in a general sense: "Whatever you propose to do, based on common sense, will almost inevitably make matters worse rather than better. You cannot meddle with one part of a complex system without the almost certain risk of setting off disastrous events that you hadn't counted on in other, remote parts. . . . Intervening is a way of causing trouble." I always think of a swinging door—the more you push in one direction, the bigger rebound you get.

A basic but lamentable ignorance is at work here. People who want control see reality as an entirely linear progression: success after success. Because of their emotional investment in their own success, they cannot entertain the notion that life in general is not like this, but rather a cyclical affair consisting of peaks and valleys. They want all of life to be peaks, but of course life can't and won't continue at this pace, on any level. Gregory Bateson has observed, again and again, that the individual creature *must* be bound by the characteristics of the overall system in which he is embedded. As Chapter 4 mentioned, the alternating rhythm of excitement and inhibition is the fundamental property of nerve cells; a little rest is always required between firings. People who make all of their life the equivalent of "firing" are in for trouble; in fact, I have argued that addiction of all types is the body's way of forcing torpor on a creature whose ideas prevent him from resting properly. As Bateson says, "To *want* control is the pathology, not that the person gets control because of course you never do."

Any individual life is a process, and any individual act within that life is a smaller process. People who want control over things don't understand process, probably because it implies the notion of something working *itself* out. Control-loving people who measure their successes only by quantity also can't stand the thought of making errors, although trial and error is the heart of any learning process. If you were doing a jigsaw puzzle, you would know intuitively that the sensible way to proceed was to patiently fit lots and lots of pieces together wrong, thus discovering which ones *did* fit. But dieters have never understood that this is what makes sense for losing weight. The Type A mind-set, coupled with an overwhelming dissatisfaction with one's present body, makes it impossible to feel that one has the leisure to make any errors. So, paradoxically, trying to do it "fast," we never learn how to do it "right," and thus spend our lives in one failure after another. As Lewis Thomas writes, "Mistakes are at the very base of human thought, embedded there, feeding the structure like root nodules. If we were not provided with the knack of being wrong, we could never get anything useful done. We think our way along by choosing between right and wrong alternatives." After quarreling with the word *error* as used in *trial and error* (because it makes this basically exploratory process sound as if it contained an element of mistake), Thomas concludes, "Biology needs a better word than 'error' for the driving force in evolution. Or maybe 'error' will do after all, when you remember that it came from an old root meaning to wander about, looking for something."

A cybernetic view of problem-solving shows us that to "accept" is a much better attitude than to "control." As Ira Progoff wisely remarked in a workshop, "Sometimes life's deepest problems are not amenable to direct assault." We may be convinced of this at least in part by physiological concerns—for example, the influence of hormones on our emotions and behavior.

No matter what the source, we need continuous reminders of these truths. Exactly such reminders are at the heart of the great body of meditative and contemplative literature from both Eastern and Western traditions. The rest of this chapter is an attempt to synthesize wisdom from several sources in the literature of "not-trying": Christianity, Buddhism, meditative athletics, systems theory. My purpose is to demonstrate the fundamental resemblances among disciplines whose diversity of metaphor may obscure the basic similarity of message. If one discipline or thinker talks about "God," another speaks of "circuits," and a third mentions "mindfulness," it may be hard to understand that they are all referring to the same idea or principle. To some it may seem blasphemous to link "sacred" subjects with systems theory or cell physiology, but without vivifying connections such as these our grasp of the fundamental truth of religious assertions is less securely founded.

Zen is perhaps the best-known philosophical formulation (insofar as it can be spoken of that way) of the illusoriness of effort. Zen literature provides a serene sense of how to live life peacefully without trying. The epigraph to this chapter aptly represents the overall spirit of Suzuki's *Zen Mind, Beginner's Mind*. Elsewhere in that volume he says, "To give your sheep or cow a large, spacious meadow is the way to control him." With respect to making errors he reports, "One continuous mistake can also be Zen.... We say, 'A good father is not a good father.' Do you understand? One who thinks he is a good father is not a good father; one who thinks he is a good husband is not a good husband."

My book frequently notes the particular relevance of Timothy Gallwey's Inner Game books to the problem at hand. More than any other individual, Gallwey has popularized and Westernized meditative ideas and—better yet—adapted them for use in action, a sort of athletic biofeedback. Gallwey comments, "It does take *effort* to run across the court and hit a tennis ball, but it does not take *trying*." He says that we need to relinquish the attempt to control ourselves by means of Self 1, the carping, self-critical part of our mind. With Self 1 distracted and occupied elsewhere, we can trust the body to do whatever is being done (play tennis, ski, etc.) to the best of its natural ability. Gallwey's axioms are: trust the body; quiet the mind; increase awareness of what is.

The Inner Game books are useful no matter what the endeavor at hand. But compulsive people need references more directly applicable to their particular problem—writings that deal specifically with the relation between addictive behavior and the philosophy of "not-trying." Gregory Bateson's essay "The Cybernetics of 'Self': A Theory of Alcoholism," which appears in *Steps to an Ecology of Mind*, clarifies many issues of addiction better than any previous work. Bateson sees alcoholics as extreme examples of the incorrect outlook characteristic of Western culture; to him, alcoholics that recover through the strenuous spiritual regime of Alcoholics Anonymous do so because they have acquired a more effective personal belief system. Bateson argues,

If [the alcoholic's] style of sobriety drives him to drink, then that style must contain error or pathology; and intoxication must provide some—at least subjective—correction of this error....

The friends and relatives of the alcoholic commonly urge him to be "strong" and to "resist temptation." What they mean by this is not very clear, but it is significant that the alcoholic himself—while sober—commonly agrees with their view of his "problem." . . . [AA does not regard alcoholics who cannot admit that they are "powerless over alcohol" as promising]; their despair is inadequate and after a more or less brief spell of sobriety they will again attempt to use "self-control" to fight the "temptation." They will not or cannot accept the premise that, drunk or sober, the total personality of an alcoholic is an alcoholic personality which cannot conceivably fight alcoholism.

One section of Bateson's essay is titled "Alcoholic 'Pride'," which refers to "an obsessive acceptance of a challenge, a repudiation of the proposition 'I cannot.' " To recover from alcoholism, the addict must first be disabused of this notion: "To be defeated by the bottle and to know it is the first 'spiritual experience.' The myth of self-power is thereby broken by the demonstration of a greater power. . . . Philosophically viewed, this first step is *not* a surrender; it is simply a change in epistemology, a change in how to know about the personality-in-the-world." Bateson makes an explicit link between religious ideas and systems theory, stating that "the theology of Alcoholics Anonymous coincides closely with an epistemology of cybernetics." As I mentioned in the previous chapter, the dilemma is that the compulsive people who suffer from various addictions such as alcoholism or overeating are those who are most unable to accept a serene view of the world; the thoughts they are thinking are the result of (among other things) their biochemical makeup. But every circle of cause and effect can be broken somewhere; for those whose despair is profound enough to jolt them out of their old ways, change is possible.

Alcoholics Anonymous literature itself provides the most eloquent statement possible of the bankruptcy of the "I can, I will" philosophy of control (which AA calls "an extreme example of self-will run riot") and the hope for recovery by means of a totally different mental orientation. The first three crucial steps of the AA program are as follows:*

1. We admitted we were powerless over alcohol—that our lives had become unmanageable.

* Quotations from Alcoholics Anonymous literature have been used throughout this book because AA is the source of most of the written materials used by related "Anonymous" programs. Overweight people should be aware, however, of the existence of Overeaters Anonymous, an organization whose principles are identical to the AA program. For further information write Overeaters Anonymous World Service Office, 2190 190th Street, Torrance, California 90504.

2. Came to believe that a Power greater than ourselves could restore us to sanity.
3. Made a decision to turn our will and our lives over to the care of God *as we understood Him.*

Twelve Steps and Twelve Traditions declares:

It was only at the end of a long road, marked by successive defeats and humiliations, and the final crushing of our self-sufficiency, that we began to feel humility as something more than a condition of groveling despair. . . . To get completely away from our aversion to the idea of being humble, to gain a vision of humility as the avenue to true freedom of the human spirit, to be willing to work for humility as something to be desired for itself, takes most of us a long, long time.

The usefulness of defeat is known to other disciplines as well. The Zen master traditionally gives his disciple a koan (a paradoxical problem like "What is the sound of one hand clapping?"). The obedient disciple revolves the problem in his mind, trying to solve it with the only tool he knows—his rational mind. He becomes more and more frustrated at his inability to *do* what it takes to solve it (in other words, his performance anxiety increases to an unbearable level), until at some point his ego cracks and in despair he gives up the attempt. At this humbling moment wisdom is born, and he gains a new intuitive insight into reality. Religious people would say he had had a conversion experience; brain physiologists would say that entirely new neuron pathways had been created.

The metaphor used to describe the experience is more or less irrelevant; only its effect upon the mind matters. Understanding this, we would be able to see that Step Three of the "Anonymous" programs is not a statement about a concept called "God" as much as a statement about the willingness to "let go." It is an issue not of belief as much as of a quality of being. In *The Crack in the Cosmic Egg* Joseph Chilton Pearce defines the conversion experience as essentially a mental reorientation: *"Metanoia* is the Greek word for conversion: a 'fundamental transformation of mind.' . . . Formerly associated with religion, *metanoia* proves to be the way by which all genuine education takes place. . . . To be *converted* is to be seized by an idea that orients us around a single focal point of possibility. . . . Conversion is like a laser; it centers the diffusing and fragmented energy into a tight, potent focus."

What we're really searching for is not the latest weight-loss technique, or indeed for anything to do with weight loss alone. What we're after is a new way to see the world, an alteration of perspective that will change the way the world looks to us forever. To quote the "Big Book" of Alcoholics Anonymous: "Unless this person can experience an entire psychic change there is very little hope of his recovery. . . . Once a psychic change has occurred, the very same person who seemed doomed . . . suddenly finds himself easily able to control his desire for alcohol, the only effort necessary being that required to follow a few simple rules."

To people accustomed to control the notion of a life based on humility is scarcely appealing. The remainder of this chapter will try to describe the benefits to be gained from emptying oneself of self-importance, realizing that, as the Zen parable says, it is only the empty vessel that can be filled.

Bateson would say that one gives up control to exist harmoniously within the confines of the whole system. As Don Juan says in Castaneda's *Tales of Power,* "When we decide, all we're doing is acknowledging that something beyond our understanding has set up the frame of our so-called decision, and all we do is to acquiesce." In the previous chapter I argued that discipline should not be seen as self-denial but rather as a willing self-fulfillment. That definition needs further amplification: discipline is a matter not of controlling oneself but of relinquishing the notion of control. George Leonard quotes the mystical golf instructor Shivas Irons of Michael Murphy's *Golf in the Kingdom* as saying, "You are a lucky man if you can find a strong beautiful discipline, one that takes you beyond yourself."

Closely allied with the concept of discipline is that of discipleship; *discipline* and *disciple* come from the same root. The humility required for a journey of discipleship is balanced perfectly with the satisfaction of being in relationship. Diet books are coming to share this notion of the joys of discipline-within-relationship. In *From Fat to Skinny,* for example, Reich spoke of the invaluable encouragement he received from a "Trusted Other"—in his case a sympathetic, understanding woman friend. A short but enlightening book, Jansen and Catlett's *The Love Diet Strategy,* is based wholly on this idea: throughout the weight loss period the dieter's food is chosen by a trusted friend, who provides both sympathy and direction. The authors aver that a great deal of a compulsive eater's resistance to change can be traced to a chronic sense of isolation coupled with a basic distrust of other people. By means of their method, notions of relationship and commitment come to predominate over self-indulgence—or, as they say, "Friendship now [comes] first instead of food." The success of the effort will be directly related to the quality of the relationship; thus it would undoubtedly be more desirable to depend on a sympathetic, loving friend rather than on a distant or condescending medical "expert."

Being part of a satisfying relationship can make it much easier to sustain disciplined serenity and focus in one's life. Interestingly enough, even compulsive people who abhor the notion of relinquishing self-control normally have access in their sex lives to a highly intense form of the benefits of the meditative state of mind—loss of self, merging with another, fascinated attention to the present moment. Unfortunately, for some especially rigid people sex is the *only* way they ever allow themselves to lapse from self-control.

Fairy tales and folk tales abound with accounts of the journey toward enlightenment in which the characters ignorantly search for gifts, only to find that the journey itself—its events, its relationships— bestowed them. *The Wizard of Oz* is like that, as is the story of the frog and the princess. The frog can only turn into the handsome prince by means of the relationship with the princess, whose unself-conscious concern for him *as he is* can release him from his enchantment. May it happen to each of us.

9
Your Own Personal Universe

Our experience shapes our perception, yet our experiences are different. So what is it that's real out there? Does the world have vertical stripes or horizontal stripes? It depends on the paradigm.

Adam Smith, *Powers of Mind*

So many people see obesity as a Problem that no one thinks to look at it as a problem—like a problem in solid geometry or trigonometry. To "solve a problem" means only to exercise mental faculties in search of a solution at present unknown; it emphatically does *not* mean to feel anxious about the problem or suffer guilt over it. Chapter 8 argued that many personal problems—obesity among them—exist in a self-perpetuating cybernetic universe. Thus to solve the problem, the question of what to do is secondary to the issue of *how to see*. The task of this chapter is to define the nature of human perception so as to make clear that it is indeed an active, not a passive, human problem-solving faculty.

In his latest book, *The Sense of Order,* E. H. Gombrich observes that "all perception is a working hypothesis to establish a fit between our senses and the reality of the outside world." Perception is not static; it is very much an ongoing cybernetic process that results in a universe tailored to the needs of each perceiver. Each of us is a goal-seeking mechanism that receives constant feedback (in the form of sense impressions) to inform us about ourselves from moment to moment.

Feedback is the constantly arriving data from which our private universe is constructed. Norbert Wiener, the father of cybernetics, gives the following formal definition of feedback: "a continual improvement of performance on the basis of past experience." (This is, of course, also the definition of trial and error.) According to Wiener, the pattern for the desired action exists; the difference between the pattern and the motion performed is used as a new input, to move the action closer to the pattern. Dr. Maxwell Maltz phrases the same idea slightly differently: "The Actual Self is necessarily imperfect. Throughout life it is always *moving toward* an ideal goal, but never arriving. It is never completed and final, but always in a state of growth."

We think we know the goal we are seeking fairly well: to lose weight, of course. However, unknown to us our bodyminds may be seeking a goal that is exactly the opposite of what we had in mind. For example, take the advice frequently found in diet books: go out and buy a dress several sizes too small and hang it up where you can see it all the time. This will provide motivation. From the point of view of cybernetic feedback, this is nonsense. When you buy yourself the smaller dress you probably send a message to your body that it is unacceptable *right now;* as long as you keep worriedly comparing your present body with the dress to the former's disadvantage, you will have set up a condition of enough anxiety that you will practically have to overeat in order to comfort yourself.

We are a collection of messages we send ourselves, which form a set of self-fulfilling predictions. Our brains are inundated with sense data every moment of our lives; we wouldn't be able to function if we had to pay close attention to everything we happened to encounter. So our brain begins to impose a pattern on reality, formed from our earlier learning experiences. We gain the ability to manipulate and interpret the things we *do* perceive, but only by losing the things our brain has chosen *not* to perceive. Each of us is thus an instrument tuned to receive only certain channels; our perception is highly selective. Some of our perceptive biases are cultural; others personal. But no sensory experience escapes selection and interpretation.

We look at the world as if through a patterned pane of glass, though we have become habituated to the pattern and no longer know it's there. In *Powers of Mind* Adam Smith spoke of "stepping outside the paradigm" in order to understand that we are always inside one. Joseph Chilton Pearce quotes Nietzsche as saying that "we hear only the question to which we are capable of finding an answer." Pearce continues: "A question to which we can respond with a full investment of life and energy will influence our 'editorial hierarchy' of mind. Then the kind of data we *accept* as *evidential* will be different. We will screen out and let in, interpret and synthesize, on a different basis." Our perceptive biases tell us what we think is "real" or "the truth"—all data that don't fit that prior definition are simply discarded.

Because we receive data from our surroundings constantly, the dimensions of our personal universe are nothing more than the sum of the messages we accept—that is, choose to pay attention to, whether consciously or subliminally. But if that is true, how can we know what criteria we have employed to choose things to attend to or to discard?

The selection process is exceedingly simple: the messages we retain are those that have some new information relative to a goal we're trying to pursue. In other words, the definition of feedback still applies. All the information that we permit into our perceptive universe is being allowed in because it's going to help us *improve our performance,* no matter what the performance is. The performance can be virtuoso whining, or it can be accomplishment—it makes no difference; the only thing that counts is that we will continue to get better and better at whatever we've chosen to pursue. Unfortunately, however, we may unconsciously choose an overall life goal, then continue to accept feedback that advances that goal in an ongoing fog of incomprehension. Feedback is a "given" in life; it is imperative that we develop an awareness of it and a sophistication in manipulating it for our benefit instead of to our detriment.

The opinions we choose to hold about ourselves are also an inevitable end product of selective perception. Once we've decided something about ourselves (that we're ugly, say), our perceptive mechanisms allow us to notice only the experiences that confirm that opinion. Soon we are "practicing" (getting better and better at) that feeling. In fact, many weight-loss strategies in diet books unwittingly provide practice for obese people to get better and better at being fat people! Later in this chapter and in Chapter 12 I will discuss ways to break out of this kind of self-defeating mind-set.

So why choose to practice thinking about yourself as fat and ugly? One might argue that fat people aren't the only ones who think they're ugly; other people do, too, and fat people can't change the way other people feel about them. Granted, this culture is not hospitable to the overweight. But the point is that if you are on the receiving end of criticism that hurts your feelings, you must have agreed with that evaluation beforehand or it would have sounded no more hurtful than a string of nonsense syllables. Of course, it isn't true (as the children's jingle goes) that words can *never* hurt me, but if they do hurt they've got to be words I've already used on myself often enough to believe that they're true.

Chapter 4 demonstrated that the equilibrium, or homeostasis, your body will seek and strive to maintain is ultimately controlled by a larger idea: who you think you are. There is a certain automatic quality to all this. Joseph Chilton Pearce quotes H. H. Price: "An idea or response tends to fulfill itself or execute itself automatically through the muscular apparatus of the body, and will do so unless other ideas are present to inhibit it." If you keep practicing thoughts of being fat, ugly, and unacceptable, then that's the kind of body you will have.

I can already hear the rebuttal: "But what am I supposed to *do?* Right now I *am* fat, ugly, and unattractive. Surely you don't want me to deny reality altogether; people who do that get locked up in asylums." That argument begs the question. My point is that a beneficial state of mind is the *sine qua non* for any meaningful change in the body. You have to be able to make that imaginative leap into how it would feel if you *were* thin before you can hope to make that experience a reality. As Dr. Maxwell Maltz explains, "You cannot merely imagine a new self-image unless you feel that it is based upon *truth*. Experience has shown that when a person does change his self-image, he has the feeling that for one reason or another, he 'sees' or realizes the truth about himself. . . . It is the function of the automatic mechanism to supply the 'means whereby' when you supply the goal."

Chapter 3 mentioned the Gestalt perception theory concepts of figure and ground—the former being whatever stands out in relief and the latter being everything else, a kind of featureless background not differentiated by the perceiver. *Ground* is that which no longer sends any new information to the brain; it's whatever you already know you know, so to speak. Habituation is the mechanism by which things that may have once been figure become ground: as you learn enough about something, you know it automatically and no longer need to pay attention to it. The furnishings of my office have become ground to me, though if the rug were changed overnight, I would certainly perceive it as figure the next day. Paradoxically, whatever is ground in your personal universe is that way for one of two diametrically opposite reasons: either you were never interested in it enough to perceive it at all, or you are so familiar with it that it has become a part of you, encoded in your synapses. For this reason our own evaluation of how conscious we are of something is not a highly reliable source. If I said, "Oh, I never think about that at all," the statement could be true in two senses. Either it is irrelevant to me, or it is so much ingrained that it "thinks me" rather than vice versa.

All new experiences are figure just because they have so much new about them to be absorbed, a fact which can explain many puzzles connected with the way we know and react to things. One of the most curious of these is the placebo effect, the well-known fact that people can sometimes be healed of a physical complaint merely by being told that the medication they are taking (which could be only a sugar pill) will help them. For years doctors have thought of the placebo effect as evidence of the mindless gullibility of their patients, though it is actually a verifiable demonstration of the awesome powers of the human bodymind. Maltz writes, "To write off placebos as 'merely due to suggestion' explains nothing. More reasonable is the conclusion that in taking the 'medicine' some sort of expectation of improvement is aroused, a goal-image of health is set up in the mind, and the creative mechanism works through the body's own healing mechanism to accomplish the goal."

Another example of this kind of seizure of the bodymind by an entirely new, positive idea is the one I mentioned in Chapter 2: losing weight effortlessly when one is in love. When it first happened to me, it seemed a mysterious side effect of the infatuation, but now it seems only inevitable. What happens when you fall in love? First, your lover seems nearly perfect to you, which makes the universe seem highly agreeable, which in turn makes it easy to sustain thankful (that is, stress-free) feelings. Next, you have something utterly fascinating to focus your attention on totally. You give up hanging around asking yourself, "When can I eat next?" You simply eat less because, temporarily, eating will nearly disappear from your perceptive universe; there are much more important things on your mind. If the attraction is mutual, your lover will be sending you constant messages that you are perfect in his or her eyes. You wouldn't think of questioning the judgment of such a perfect person, and soon you will begin to feel wonderful about yourself, too. Your bodymind will begin to act upon these suggestions as instructions, making you into someone as perfect as it is possible for you to be—to the limits of your imagination. In *The Body Clock Diet,* Dr. Ronald Gatty observes, "In my experience, there is a curious fact about women: if they fall in love, they can lose weight with phenomenal ease and rapidity no matter what kind of food you put in front of them."

There is also a cybernetic explanation for another puzzling phenomenon, the paradoxical short-lived potency of posthypnotic suggestion. A hypnotist could suggest to a hypnotized client that he or she would not want to overeat after leaving the session. The client would probably find (to his or her utter amazement) that this was true—but only for about three days. Why? If the effect was strong enough at first to overturn well-established habits, why couldn't it last? The suggestion was not only new, but also given under hypnosis, a state of hyperattention. The bodymind accepted the suggestion and started to work on it. But we are basically information-processing systems, and new data are always arriving. If the suggestion did not fit seamlessly into the client's established goal-seeking personal universe (and if it had, of course, he or she wouldn't have been seeking help with his or her "problem"), without further reinforcement it would have been supplanted by others more necessary to the maintenance of his or her familiar universe.

Think of "Cinderella" as a cybernetic tale. Cinderella is the archetypal female who sees herself as deserving a pitiful and unsatisfying fate. Gifts of ego enhancement and beneficial feedback arrive unexpectedly (the Fairy Godmother and the pretty clothes). Cinderella accepts them eagerly and goes off to the ball. But without an internal source of perpetuating the complimentary feedback, she must lose them at midnight. We all process data constantly, and good suggestions from outside often get crowded out by the demands of our more familiar negative self-concept. Men who can't identify with Cinderella's plight might ponder "Beauty and the Beast," also a cybernetic fable.

A friend of mine once startled me by musing, "Every diet only works once, doesn't it?" She was right. The first time on any diet the placebo effect is at work; you're willing to invest all your belief and expectation that this one will do the job—and it *does*. If, as frequently happens, you later gain the weight back, the diet loses some of its magic in your eyes; you can use it again, but never in that same spirit of wholehearted acceptance. When your critical self takes over in subsequent tries, the placebo effect vanishes and you find it impossible to get the same results.

Obese people live in a very interesting perceptual universe; for them the "problem" of their obesity will forever be figure—something to always notice and constantly agonize over. On the other hand, unwise eating habits—all the *experiences* that constitute the *process* that is obesity—very quickly become ground, and hence totally unavailable for conscious examination. The great value of behavior modification techniques for overweight people is allowing them to see accurately, perhaps for the first time, exactly what it is they do. Once aware, many can change their habits with surprising rapidity.

Aversion conditioning could also be helpful, if only because it breaks up the habituated identification of certain foods with "deliciousness." In his new book *Mind and Nature* Gregory Bateson speaks of the folly of thinking that the object "out there" contains some explanatory principle or characteristic. Bateson posits the *relationship* between a substance and its user as the only concept of any importance. Overweight people are very prone to ascribe their lack of will power to the "deliciousness" of the available food. However, the food's deliciousness for you originates in some decisions about your relation to food made long before any specific temptation shows up.

Certain types of experiences seem to be permanently exempted from becoming ground. When we define a certain class of experiences as interesting to us, each new instance will always call itself to our attention. If we are learning things in a new field, for example, we will be sensitized to any new item of information we happen to encounter. If we are collectors of something—wines, antiques, or the like—we will notice any novel items we run across. Or basic drives may provide the necessary impetus: most men react to each female they find attractive with undiminished interested attention. Hunger is another basic drive, normally of a cyclical nature: people who eat according to their body signals will be highly aware of the existence of food when they are hungry, but much less interested when they are not. This criterion divides obese mind-set eaters from normal eaters; the former have been called *data-driven* because they react with appetite to the mere presence of food, not to hunger cues from their bodies. Beller cites one remarkable experiment showing that overweight people ate about as much as a control group of normal people when extra helpings were out of sight and slightly difficult to obtain, but up to three times as much as the normal eaters when the extra helpings were already present on the plate.

Certain other perceptions never become ground because they are habitually experienced in an altered state of consciousness like self-hypnosis. Susan Newton told me that an overeater is someone who is so suggestible to the sight of food that he or she goes into a type of self-induced hypnotic trance and eats too much—in fact, with no stop cues whatever—without conscious awareness of doing so. In an article called "Fat Control," Amy Gross once facetiously characterized herself as a person who "goes into a trance and comes to with an empty box of cookies in hand and crumbs on her fingers."

But hypnosis is any kind of hyperattention, anything we've agreed to pay closer than usual attention to. Maltz says, "Every human being is hypnotized to some extent, either by ideas he has uncritically accepted from others, or ideas he has repeated to himself or convinced himself are true." Unfortunately, we are highly vulnerable to being hypnotized by negative things other people think and say about us (because we're so prone to believe the worst about ourselves). If you are making a sincere effort to lose weight, yet feel sabotaged by someone's hurtful criticism, you will have to realize, first, that *you* are giving the criticism whatever significance it has for you. Then you may have to take some common-sense action, such as avoiding that person during the time you are losing weight. On the other hand, the opposite problem can also exist, as I can testify. I was once so hypersensitive to criticism that I ascribed to my husband disgusted, critical thoughts I later discovered he wasn't even thinking (a marvelous example of one's ability to generate purely imaginary feedback for the purposes of self-torture).

This may be the place to talk about supportive feedback from one's spouse. A woman who's been married thirty years may well reply, "My husband loves me and I know it. But just knowing it doesn't seem to help me do anything about my weight." This is a good example of habituation at work: the wife's "knowledge" that her husband loves her is based on the fact that it's always been that way. However, his love for her has also become so predictable that she can no longer pick up any new vitalizing messages from it. She must take the initiative, looking for ways to help *herself* feel new feelings of being desired and cherished, arranging all the familiar information their marriage contains into new patterns of meaning. When she has a new sense of desirability, she will unconsciously communicate this to her spouse, whose response will probably be encouraging. It could be the beginning of a new self-fulfilling circle of mutual appreciation.

In *Cybernetics* Wiener observes of cybernetic feedback in general, "We often find a message contaminated by extraneous disturbances which we call *background noise*." With personal feedback, anxiety and self-criticism are the background noise. Maltz claims, "When excessive negative feedback, or self-criticism, was eliminated, inhibition disappeared and performance improved." We all tend to identify with our most negative self-evaluation, though that is pointless. Richard Hittleman writes in his *Guide to Yoga Meditation,*

> Imagine a television set on which the switch is broken so that you cannot turn it off. You sit and watch the programs endlessly until there comes a time when you forget that there ever was an "off" switch. That is what has happened in the case of our ordinary minds. We let the thoughts run on endlessly, hour after hour, day after day, year after year, giving them our full attention and energy until we forget that they are simply facts, statistics, being played over and over like a phonograph record.

Bateson repeatedly stresses that all meaning is a function of context. Now that we have spent so much time on the individual's personal cybernetic context, it is time to consider the operation of larger cybernetic universes. We have seen the redundant mechanisms by which homeostasis is preserved in the body; for a person to be obese, he must be doing obesity-producing activities on several levels simultaneously. The world at large works the same way. Everything that is a constant feature of our life is there because its existence is underwritten in several separate and redundant ways. We exist in several overlapping contexts at once: as a separate person, as a participant in close relationships, and as a member of a culture. In each of these universes we are the sum of the messages we accept and act on.

Obesity consciousness can (in fact, nearly *must*) be mutually reinforcing in more than one context. People who dislike themselves for being fat may also find themselves in relationships with people who are either overtly critical or misguidedly "trying to help" with the problem. In addition, of course, we are members of the most obesity-conscious culture in the history of the human race. Thus there are nested contexts and mutually encouraging agreed-upon ways to think of oneself and behave. This notion of multiple contexts in which you stay fat may sound pessimistic. However, the consolation is that the only level that *truly matters* is the personal; get your own universe in order, and you can gain the necessary perspective on how to resolve the others.

Chapters 13 and 14 will go into greater detail about feedback connected with dieting itself. Recording your food intake, making a weight chart, writing your feelings in a journal, keeping an exercise log are all feedback tools, helping to foster awareness of what you do and providing a gauge of your progress as you go. But the greatest possible sophistication is required in order to elicit genuine, intelligible feedback from your dieting. Only truthful, not spurious, feedback can provide guidance for improved action as well as encouragement rather than despair. The essence of feedback is measurement, or sampling: you need to choose the right progress measures and the right intervals for checking them. Measuring the wrong things, or measuring too frequently, can cloud the pattern that is there or even obscure it altogether. Men can always get more rational answers from the scale than women, since they do not share either women's complex hormonal interplay or their periodic water retention problems.

In addition, you must develop enough sensitivity to the rhythms and pattern of your own process that you don't try to forcefully extract feedback that isn't suitable or informative. For example, no matter what the diet, the loss of fat occurs so slowly it is invisible to any measurement device. (It is like the hour hand on the clock—you can only see that it *has* moved, not that it *is* moving.) Dieters who use a daily weigh-in on the bathroom scale as their index of progress are unwittingly relying on the previous day's loss of water to shore up their self-esteem, since only water enters and leaves the body rapidly enough and in large enough quantities to be visible on the scale from one day to the next. And if an exercise program were adding to the person's muscle mass, a well-behaved dieter could actually get on the scale and find a weight *gain* (as heavier muscle tissue substitutes for the fat). Without sophistication in the interpretation of what the feedback means, the dieter would feel discouraged for no good reason.

Dieters who have set deadlines for themselves based on the conventional wisdom about how long it takes to lose a certain amount of weight can only be happy at the very beginning of their diet, when large amounts of water are lost with the standard amount of fat. Toward the end of the diet, when there isn't as much water left to be lost, the same fat loss (which in actuality has remained constant throughout) now seems unacceptably slow, the cause for a great deal of self-recrimination. It would be much more sensible to use as a feedback tool one's diminishing *size* over the dieting period, since this more accurately reflects fat loss and is less subject to the erratic ups and downs of numbers on the scale.

A change in *how to see* that precedes one's understanding of the right actions to reach the goal can be sudden and permanent. It is like shaking the kaleidoscope: one moment there was one pattern, and the next moment—*out of the same materials*—another prettier pattern has assembled itself. To acquire this new perceptive universe, first become exquisitely aware of all the messages you presently hear with your inner ear and then unconsciously act on. Second, use awareness tools (see the next chapter) to become highly sensitized in totally new areas; you can learn to focus intently upon, or even become hypnotized by, whole classes of new experiences other than food. Chapter 12 goes into much greater detail about how to implement new goals, but the basic principles are these: every sensory experience in a dieter's life should provide pleasant, joyful feedback so that the bodymind—the part that actually works on the goal—can perform its tasks with a minimum of distractions or obstacles. Learn to control that for yourself and you will have the most powerful tool possible at your command.

Cybernetics provides a new way of judging the success of your problem-solving efforts—that is, when you succeed, the problem disappears from consciousness. When the learning you have needed to do to reach your goal is complete, and a new perceptual universe has been shaken from the remnants of the old, insofar as your new reality does what you specified, it will become habituated and unremarkable. It makes a lot of sense, actually: naturally thin people just go about being thin without needing to comment on what's happening—it isn't a problem, it isn't an issue, it's simply absent from their perceptive universe. When you *have* a problem, you need to think about it a lot and work on strategies to solve it; when you *don't* have a problem, none of that is required. Anything you still think you have to work at "controlling," you haven't sufficiently learned. You will know you've solved your problem when you don't have to think about it any more, for the simple reason that you have made your way into the ranks of normally thin people. This is the only possible definition of having arrived.

10
Learning through Awareness

We never look enough, never exactly enough, never passionately enough.

Colette, *Paris from My Window*

In this chapter *awareness* is used to denote a mental condition that fosters the ability to learn new things. Later chapters will be more specific about the kinds of things a dieter has to learn in order to start losing weight, but for the moment we need to focus on the learning process itself in order to discover which of our culturally determined mental habits hinder us from learning new things and which can be used to help us.

Recent studies of the human brain reveal that we learn things in ways we never suspected when we were struggling with the multiplication tables back in the fourth grade. Learning occurs ceaselessly every moment of a person's waking life. It consists of the experiences our body is having, often but not necessarily mediated by the conscious mind's interpretation of those experiences. When the results of this kind of learning are communicated to the learner, it is called biofeedback. Barbara Brown commented to an interviewer, "Biofeedback is a learning process. I happen to believe that the biofeedback learning phenomenon is quite a different kind of learning from any that has ever been defined in academia, and no existing theories explain it at all well."

Learning is not something that only our conscious mind does. Since we are conscious only of our conscious mind, we believe that it is the agent that does everything for us. However, this is an illusion just as fallacious as the apparent truth that the sun goes around the earth. The truth is that the learning is done by the entire bodymind, the unconscious as well as the conscious. Barbara Brown tells us in *New*

Mind, New Body that every square inch of our body contains innumerable receptors for sense data: "The mindbody bristles with receiver sets, like banks of radar and sonar sensors. Its antennae are not only the eyes and ears and skin-touching receivers; mind-body is affected by temperature, magnetic fields, love and kindness, being ignored or misled, by vibrations, physical and emotional. Mind-body is an omnivorous harvester of information." She reports the following fascinating experiment which proved that the body "knows" things independently of conscious awareness:

Naughty words or other emotion-arousing words were flashed on a screen so briefly that the subjects could not perceive them intelligently.... Although it was impossible for the subjects to see the words and so consciously recognize them, something in their brains *did* recognize every word, and this recognition was voiced by the skin. For every naughty word there was an orienting response by the skin, but no responses to the neutral or bland words.

What does it mean to say that learning is carried out by the entire bodymind in ways we may not be fully aware of? As experiments in brain physiology have recently shown, the two hemispheres of the brain have very different characteristics: the left hemisphere processes and interprets words, while the right hemisphere processes our wordless experiences—images, sensory data, and the like. Since both halves of the brain are doing the learning, our bodymind learns as much from wordless sense data as from words. In fact, recent discoveries indicate the right hemisphere may be more useful than the left as a problem-solving tool.

The old saying "I'm sorry, but who you are speaks so clearly I can't hear what you're saying" describes perfectly the way the bodymind works, capturing the nuances of a given situation so that we can experience it as a (wordless) unity. The trouble is, however, that we are so word-infatuated in this culture that we simply don't trust anything that doesn't know how to talk, even though many of our most accurate perceptions are received as pictorial images by the right hemisphere of the brain. If we want to converse with our bodyminds, however, we will simply have to accept the fact that they don't speak English; talking to them requires becoming familiar with *their* language.

Because they are wordless, and we are sensitized to words, our right-brain perceptions seem subliminal, below our level of conscious awareness. Many of us may have difficulty even admitting that we perceive things subliminally, let alone learning how to become aware of them; subliminal things are, after all, by nature invisible. But just because something is not apparent to our usual level of consciousness doesn't mean that it doesn't exist, only that we don't see it. Instead of ignoring invisible things, we must lower our threshold of awareness so that the unseen things begin to appear.

How do we lower our awareness threshold? First, by quieting the chatter of our Outer Self so that we have more of our attention available for close, accurate perception. We need to transfer our faith from the "I" that once seemed responsible for our problem solving to the process itself—in other words, to the way things unfold and become clearer "all by themselves." Wilfred Barlow's book about body awareness, *The Alexander Technique,* makes this statement: "We too often make this mistake of *doing* some fixed thing, instead of engaging in some process; we *read, copulate, eat, speak,* instead of engaging in the *process* of reading, the *process* of copulation, the *process* of eating, the *process* of speaking. . . . When we are concerned with *ends* rather than *means,* our bodies don't function as well. The human organism is built for process operation, not for end-gaining."

Because awareness consists of learning to see things we couldn't see before, it's obvious that what is required is to assume the role of interested observer, to develop Adam Smith's "passive volition and casual attitude." However, we in the Western world simply aren't used to being passive; we persist in the belief that to achieve anything, in any field whatever, we have to be trying. Biofeedback technicians operating a stress-reduction program for executives reported that the first session was invariably hard on all participants, since most executives couldn't even grasp the notion of doing something whose essence was learning and making progress through not-trying. Someone accustomed to striving might wonder whether he is "really learning" anything with this seemingly lackadaisical approach. The answer is that it is impossible to *stop* learning; we learn every moment of our lives, but without awareness we often get involved in learning (and practicing) things that run counter to the goals we've set ourselves.

Knowledge one can acquire through reading; awareness is a bodily experience one can acquire only from observation. The essence of the awareness we're talking about is an increase in the quality of one's perception. To quote from Gallwey's *Inner Tennis:* "There is no learning, no growth, no action, without awareness. Awareness is the basic element of all human activities. Whatever increases it increases one's learning potential, and whatever decreases it interferes with one's learning potential. . . . There is only one way to progress in the Inner Game: to *increase awareness* of what is." In *Profound Simplicity* Will Schutz makes a similar point: "For any given situation, there is the simplest path. Awareness reveals the path. The ultimate simplicity is to choose the correct path."

We usually assume our ordinary level of perception as the given, but the truth is that—whatever our level of sensory awareness—it is only one point of a continuum ranging throughout the universe, from the minimum sensory levels of an amoeba to the highly developed sensitivities of some animals (the hearing of bats, for example). While every creature has its own somewhat fixed range of abilities, we can train ourselves to perceive much more than we now do with each of our senses and thus transcend what we think are our natural limits. Thomas Gladwin's *East is a Big Bird* tells the story of the extraordinary navigational feats accomplished by certain seafaring Micronesian tribes, who range over thousands of miles without a system of celestial navigation, using only hyperdeveloped observations of environmental features such as birds, seaweed, currents, land masses, and so forth. The author, having accompanied tribesmen on several voyages to observe their methods first-hand, comments: "In some perceptual modes, such as sensing from the direction of waves the presence of reefs below the surface, Hipour could work with discriminations I not only could not perceive but could scarcely conceive."

We have all learned to screen out an enormous amount of the sense data we receive, but it is possible to reverse this process. In any field of endeavor the truly outstanding people are those who see (that is, understand) more than others; one recalls Henry James's passionate cry, "Try to be one of the people on whom nothing is lost." Gallwey tells of seeing pretoddlers in a park intently watching children slightly older than themselves, observing with the greatest degree of concentration the exact movements required for walking upright. They were merely unself-consciously exemplifying one important precept of natural learning: that one's skill in performing any activity directly depends on how detailed was perception as one observed someone else's demonstration of the skill. For dieters the same principles apply. We have always approached learning to be thin as if it were learning the rules of grammar of a foreign language: lots of rules to memorize and lots of prohibitions. Instead, it is like learning to speak the language fluently and idiomatically: you just start doing something (with the limited abilities you have), then pay attention to your mistakes, correcting them as you perceive them, and spend time with people who know how to do what you want to do, learning from them.

Awareness, then, is basically about learning to pay much better attention. In *The Second Ring of Power,* Carlos Castaneda writes, "I knew what she had meant when she said that the art of dreamers was the art of attention." Nothing in our culture has prepared us for, or instructed us in, paying attention. In *Four Arguments for the Elimination of Television* Jerry Mander claims that television has already deleteriously affected our ability to concentrate. Each image in any given program or commercial lasts no longer than three seconds before being cut to another; thus watching television actually impairs our ability to engage in the sustained, single-pointed direction of attention that is the essence of awareness.

The kind of heightened awareness I am discussing is clearly a learned skill, a conscious and deliberate heightening of one's normal powers. Like swimming, it is not simply an innate ability; it must be learned and then practiced to achieve mastery. One's mind should become like a laser beam, gaining tremendous power through direction and focusing. Modern physiology confirms the reciprocal link between relaxation and focused awareness. R. Frank Hoffman, M.D., the instructor of a course in holistic health, explained that activating the parasympathetic nervous system (which is associated with body relaxation) brings about a sharper focus of perception; conversely, therefore, starting to focus will itself initiate the relaxation response. Focusing on *anything* is better than letting the mind continue to focus on itself, which brings on anxious thoughts and self-criticism.

It is easiest to achieve a condition of hyperawareness in the state of altered consciousness we commonly call *hypnosis.* The power of hypnosis derives from increased focus; as Dr. Herbert Spiegel of Columbia University's College of Physicians and Surgeons explained to an interviewer, "Our sense of awareness in everyday life is a constant balance between focal attention and peripheral awareness.... In a trance state you reduce your peripheral awareness and increase your focal attention." He further observes, "A hypnotic trance is a state of attentive, responsive concentration.... Not sleep. The opposite. Being aware and focused." To many people hypnosis is a loaded word meaning a sleeplike state in which one's mind is under someone else's control. "The paradox about hypnotism [says Spiegel] is what appears to be a loss of control is really an exercise in greater control." The mystical golf instructor Shivas Irons in Michael Murphy's *Golf in the Kingdom* sagely says, "Hypnosis is first cousin to fascination . . . and all art and love depend on fascination. Fascination is the true and proper mother of discipline."

To increase awareness, we need to notice that the richness of any sensory experience is inversely proportional to its speed. When concentration is very intense (as it is in hypnosis), each perceived detail is observed more closely and at greater length, which makes our subjective sense of time seem to slow down. In this culture we have become so pathologically impatient that we want to have already *finished* doing anything we're doing—particularly if that activity is losing weight. Though it would seem silly to pay for a trip abroad and then spend our every moment wishing it were already over, we don't see the foolishness of our attitudes about dieting. Losing weight is like a journey—an experience replete with learning opportunities. And, as E. B. White observed so charmingly in his *Essays,* "If our future journeys are to be little different from flashes of light, with no interim landscape and no interim thought, I think we will have lost the whole good of journeying and will have succumbed to a mere preoccupation with getting there."

We have such impatient attitudes about being overweight that we find it nearly impossible to relax about *when* we are going to get thin, though we never connect our lack of long-term success with our time-bound anxiety and dead-end methods. Losing weight is just like getting a tan. First, it takes whatever time it takes. Second, though you may want the tan very badly, if you're so ashamed of your present untanned body that you can't bear to be seen on the beach, you're in real trouble. Only being out there going through the process will get you where you want to be.

The description of perception and feedback in the last chapter stated that the two most important questions are What are you paying attention to? and, next, What does it mean? Increasing your awareness will give you a powerful tool. But it is most important to use it to increase order and coherence, and therefore extract *meaning,* and not to stop with gathering *data.* As Arthur J. Deikman observed in

Ornstein's *The Nature of Human Consciousness,* "Rather than being the product of a particular neural circuit, awareness is the *organization* of the biosystem."

Our behavior tends to be a mixture of conscious and unconscious choices: some of what we do we seem to choose, while the rest we do because we can't help it. With awareness, we can learn a great deal more about the hidden influences that produce the behavior we think we can't control. Dorelle Heisel remarks in *The Biofeedback Exercise Book,* "Behavior modification by awareness is done *by* you, not *to* you." Awareness brings you three types of knowledge or experience you couldn't get without it: (1) knowledge of behavior and feelings that the unconsciousness of habituation had formerly kept hidden from you; (2) knowledge about which of these are actually obstacles toward reaching your goals; and (3) intense present-moment experiences that, by bringing more total satisfaction into your life, reduce your need to overeat.

The first category is what I earlier called data—all the information about yourself you haven't had access to before. This information tends to group itself into the following categories: habitual eating behavior, body use and body signals, behavior in general, emotions, and relationships. There are specific books that deal in detail with each of these groups or kinds of information. Chapter 14 provides a more detailed enumeration of these.

Gathering data in each of these areas provides many surprises. As I kept records of my eating, I was astonished and dismayed to find out just how unconscious I was about how and what I ate: it took weeks and weeks of writing down every detail before I could say I knew what was going on. I'm sure I was not alone in my self-ignorance; in our culture, we often eat automatically when we see food, not as a response to biological hunger. Recent books such as *Psychological War on Fat* have labeled this behavior "robot" eating. Compulsive eating, of course, is the antithesis of awareness; it is more like anesthesia. At fast-food restaurants we can slip into Type A eating and consume thousands of calories in a matter of moments without being more than barely aware of what we've eaten.

Unfortunately, the data may provide more information than you want on behavior you feel ashamed of, although being willing to face it is the only possible path to being cured. In *Forever Thin* Dr. Rubin exhorts us to extract knowledge from binges: "It is always valuable to review the events of the hours and days immediately preceding a binge. . . . Look at a binge as a chance to extend insight rather than as an opportunity for self-hate." As Dr. Lindner used to tell his patients, "We don't consider binging a mortal sin—but not writing down what you ate certainly is."

On the other hand, it's possible that the data may vindicate the overweight person in unexpected ways. Henry Jordan et al. say in *Eating is Okay!* that "you very likely have misconceptions about fat people in general. It is a myth, for example, that they eat more food than others. Or eat more often. Or eat alone more. Our studies show that many fat people do eat a lot, and often, and alone. But so do an approximately equal number of people of normal weight."

Body awareness techniques help you break through habituated ways of perceiving and responding to your body. Thérèse Bertherat pointed out that people sometimes have stopped feeling messages from the body entirely. Overweight people need body awareness techniques because shame about the body's appearance may have led them to block out awareness of the body's feelings. As Dorelle Heisel succinctly put it, "Notice if you say, 'Not now!' when your body tells you 'I have to. . . .' " It is important to identify one's negative feelings in response to various situations, since feelings such as anger, boredom, anxiety, or resentment almost invariably serve as a cue to overeat. And as Dorothy Tennov pointed out in *Super Self,* it is useful to think of emotional responses as if they were body sensations; "this will help you pinpoint the situations that arouse [the emotion]."

There is a certain limitation to data. Although it was unquestionably better to know what my eating patterns were than to remain entirely unconscious of them, I found that I couldn't necessarily use my new knowledge to effect any meaningful change. (I must also confess at this point that I have never been able to abide those behavior modification workbook-type books that look as if they should have been printed on graph paper.) Finally I realized that the data were nothing more than an alphabet; I needed to do more work to find out what my behavior had been *saying* and what I wanted to say in its place.

In *The Meditation Diet,* Tyson and Walker even take issue with data collection itself. They contend that overeating is purely and simply a matter of attitude, and to focus on food is to miss the point entirely. "It is not a good idea to keep a food diary. The reason is simply this: . . . keeping a record of what you eat or what you do not eat turns the diet into another exercise in exaggeration. You stress dieting, and you see dieting as merely a question of the eating or non-eating of certain foods. This could tend to take you away from the idea of . . . your negative resistors as the main cause of your dietary indiscretions." I have to agree with Tyson and Walker; I found for myself that I was much better off keeping records of my feeling states at any given time, or writing a "dialogue with the body" as I learned to do in the Progoff Intensive Journal Workshop (see Chapter 14).

There is one book on food awareness, however, that satisfies my criteria for meaning: Don Gerrard's *One Bowl*. I haven't followed exactly the path outlined in his book, but it's the most sensitive description that exists of the awareness process and how to use it to change one's eating:

I eat because I am hungry but I also eat to affirm my being, my personality, my sense of life. Naturally then eating is an important emotional experience. *My diet concept begins by isolating you from external noise so that you can concentrate on your internal sounds.* Then it shows you how to interpret and evaluate these sounds for the important signals they are.

I used to eat mostly with my head, paying attention to my ideas and memories of food and to its taste, but ignoring the food once it was swallowed. Now I eat more with my whole body.

One benefit of data gathering is becoming more self-assured through increased self-knowledge. As we accumulate more genuine body experience, we can speak of ourselves with greater confidence, being, like Jung, a person who "only believes in what he knows." Even more important, awareness can make us cognizant for the first time of a larger pattern in our life, or even the pattern of all our relationships and how we fit into them. With this increased awareness of pattern, we can get a meaningful sense of cause and effect, of the complex and orderly whole.

Besides making it possible to gather formerly hidden data, the other important advantage to a life of full awareness is having our actions rescued from the unconscious, mechanical repetition which occurs in us because of habituation. With awareness each action is deliberately *chosen,* which serves to intensify the quality of experience. When each act has been consciously chosen, each is meaningful; it is this sense of meaning that keeps a discipline from seeming to be mere self-deprivation.

The discipline of behavior modification—slowing down and paying attention to our food or body signals—has its larger analogue in meditation: slowing down and paying attention to our life. Most books on meditation don't make explicit enough that awareness, like meditation, is a clearer form of perception that can also be extended to our everyday activities. Richard Hittleman's *Guide to Yoga Meditation* contains a chapter called "Experience as a Form of Meditation," which echoes a phrase in Fred Rohé's *The Zen of Running:* "from the experience of running meditatively, I learn that potentially my entire life can be lived meditatively. And it seems to me I should learn to live it so." This attitude toward life leaves us open to unexpected beauty in any experience, as Laurence Reich reported in *From Fat to Skinny:*

One morning not too long ago we found a beautiful head of Manoa lettuce. . . . It's an especially delicious variety, a leafy, deep green in color with a rich, buttery taste. To enhance the particular shade of green, we looked very carefully for carrots of just the right orange tone. Giving time and thought to these small points is a terrific way to get excited about these foods. I could hardly wait to see these vegetables on a plate.

It seems fitting to close this chapter with a quotation from *One Bowl* that describes a calm, meditative state of mind for living peacefully in one's body:

ONE BOWL has carried me into a personal way of being that is more peaceful, that allows me to detach myself from my cares and to experience myself as a whole body, a living connected being without name or desire. This is a space in which I do not know myself by thinking and do not talk to myself with words. It is a silent space, a space of pure sensation. Within it I am a biological organism; I become my body. Body sensations are my language. I live life slowly, at what I imagine to be a biochemical rate of speed, I feel immensely calm and secure. I value this space in my life enough to try to enter it at least once a day.

11
Antistress Exercises

> Meditation is not a passive process but a means of allowing an individual to enter into daily activity relatively free of neurotic distractions.
> Kenneth Pelletier, *Mind as Healer, Mind as Slayer*

Chapters 5 and 6 gave an account of what anxiety is and how it operates to the detriment of the bodymind. As I said then, anxiety fuels the overeater's central double-bind: feeling sad and guilty about being fat and therefore having to overeat in order to feel better. The next legitimate question is how to banish anxiety from your life; this chapter will provide some specific tools and insights that will help you rid yourself of this crippling, unnecessary mental disease.

The first step (a giant step, admittedly) is to learn to accept nonjudgmentally that everything in your life is—at the moment, anyway—a *given*. It just *is;* there is no right or wrong about it. As Wayne Dyer wrote in *Your Erroneous Zones,* "You are the sum total of your choices." At this moment your body is a given, too—also the inevitable result of a long series of prior choices. You are now ready to make new choices, but you can't make them as wisely and coolly if you're still full of anxious, self-blaming accusations along the lines of "Why am I so fat?" This state of mind *doesn't work,* so drop it. Self-recrimination is merely an intense dissatisfaction with *what is;* but *what is* is all that counts, all we have. Timothy Gallwey's piercing comment on the difference between *should* and *is* gets right to the heart of the issue: "The ball is seldom where it *should* be, but it is *always* where it *is.* Similarly, one must hit the ball that *is* with the racket that *is.* The racket that 'should be' will miss the ball that 'is.' 'Should' and 'is' are incompatible because they are in different dimensions."

I still remember the astonishment I felt when I heard a lecturer say, "You are exactly where you are meant to be, doing exactly what you are meant to be doing." I felt like jumping up and crying out, "I *am?*" This idea was as foreign to my usual way of seeing things as if it had been uttered in Hindustani, but in the weeks that followed it slowly, insidiously made its impression on my mind.

At this moment you may be intensely puzzled about how belief or lack of belief in the inevitability or "isness" of the present moment could possibly be connected to the attempt to relieve stress. When Dr. Hans Selye was asked if any emotion could be thought of as an antidote to stress, his response was "Yes—the attitude of thanksgiving." If you're grateful for something, you aren't simultaneously finding fault with it; an attitude of thanksgiving, in fact, goes beyond acceptance of what is to joyfully welcoming it. Obviously, happiness and joy are the opposite of anxiousness and worry; you can't feel both at the same time.

I'm not asking you to be thrilled with your excess poundage, but redressing your anxiety-induced biochemical imbalance requires that you at least accept it and do away with your customary self-hatred. Let us continue the tennis analogy for a moment. Your overeating has always been just a response to stress—the equivalent of a stroke in a tennis game, no more. You will be learning better strokes, but you don't need to deny that you ever had your old ones; they were the best you could do at the time. Trying to institute new habits should be thought of as a tennis volley. You want to keep the ball up (that is, perform impeccably) as long as possible, of course, but it's also inevitable that you will drop the ball now and then. Blaming yourself because you dropped the ball is simply foolish. I will always cherish Newman and Berkowitz's observation in *How to Be Your Own Best Friend* that people "think their choice is between being perfect and being the worst thing that ever lived."

Performance anxiety, or shame at being overweight, has at least two obvious antecedents: the tendency to take oneself too seriously or the lack of self-respect. Here's a simple test for whether or not you are taking yourself too seriously. Think of a remote acquaintance of yours who is just as overweight as you are. Do you spend an equal amount of time agonizing over his or her weight problem as you do over your own? No? Perhaps it's because you're paying yourself more (negative) attention than you really merit. Self-respect, on the other hand, is something you truly do deserve. Joan Didion observed in her essay "On Self-Respect" that this quality has nothing to do with "not having safety pins in one's underwear," nor with "the approval of others," but "concerns instead a separate peace, a private reconciliation."

Remember that you have the choice of what you'll pay attention to: your achievements or your failures. The previous chapter claimed that your life *became* what you paid the most attention to. Right now you're paying exquisitely detailed attention to the fact that you have a weight problem. Forget it! Develop a fascinated concentration on the events of your daily life instead. In terms of personal priorities, what you weigh ought to be at the bottom of your list. (I still chuckle whenever I remember Jeanne Eddy Westin's exasperated comment in *The Thin Book:* "You are not a 'weight'!") The most important item on your agenda has to be making yourself into a person who doesn't need to assuage personal difficulties by means of food.

Many people say things like "I'm so unhappy because I can't get thin." Not so. It would be more accurate in a biochemical sense to say instead, "I'm not thin because I can't get happy." Granted, being overweight *is* a problem, and it needs a solution. But anguish never brought relief. If your child were drowning, you'd be better off rescuing him instead of wringing your hands over the sadness of the whole thing. Losing weight is like that.

Psychoanalysis for obese people digs into the past to discover the way it influences present behavior. Elsewhere in this book I have glancingly dealt with the way your past influences the present, but in this chapter the past is irrelevant; all that counts is keeping your peace of mind in the *present,* because only doing that will make it unnecessary for you to overeat *now.*

The most fundamental issue is your basic state of mind; what are you choosing to be (express, practice) right now? If your answer is anything other than "calm," keep reading; you can use the help. The primary problem-solving, goal-seeking agent in our lives is the subconscious mind. Much like the Sorcerer's Apprentice, it blindly follows to the letter the instructions it has—sometimes unknowingly—been given. As Susan Newton once told me, "Your subconscious mind will create an entire universe in which what you are thinking will be useful or required." Thus if you constantly feel dissatisfied, you will continually attract into your life events that justify these feelings.

It is a difficult paradox: each of us, by having made and continuing to make choices, is totally responsible for our present life situation yet virtually powerless to influence events by means of "will power" or "trying." I wanted to think of a way to explain what sort of attitude you have to have in order to function effectively while keeping the background anxiety in your life to a minimum. As I drove down the Pacific Coast Highway, I saw the surfers riding the waves and knew that that was the analogy I had been looking for. (I later found out that John Lilly had discovered it, too, and had called it "cosmic surfing.") People who want to learn to surf just wade out in the breakers and start trying to ride *with* the waves that come crashing upon them, wave after wave after wave, without ceasing. You can't learn to surf at all if you stand out there yelling, "Why are all these damn waves happening to *me,* anyway?" and you'll get nowhere if you try to deal with them by asserting your own ego. The only way that *works* is just to *be* out there, since (1) they never stop coming; (2) they come in different sizes—some easy, some not; (3) you need to pick ones suited to your level of expertise and try to sidestep the bigger ones until they no longer overwhelm you; and (4) you need to move with them, not fight them.

Just like reality, isn't it? Every day you practice riding with the stressful events in your life while at the same time you practice keeping your inner serenity intact. In order to learn this, you have to make some mistakes, be ready to correct moves that didn't work, and *keep at it* (practice, over and over).

This chapter is not about "positive thinking." And when I speak of serenity as the desired goal, I'm not talking about an event-free life. A friend of mine once said, "So many people confuse serenity with tranquility. Tranquility is sitting all alone by a quiet mountain stream, joyfully at one with the universe. Whenever you can do that, it's great. But real serenity is the kids screaming, dinner boiling over, the washing machine broken, and you're *still* functioning. *That's* serenity."

Many more factors may be at work to keep you tense than those you're consciously aware of. In fact, as I have said earlier, the most potent and insidious stress factors in your life will be chronic and therefore subliminal. You are constantly carrying on an unspoken dialogue with your environment; you need to bring to awareness what that dialogue is saying. What we are looking for are things that make it impossible for the bodymind to relax completely. Search for cues that constantly send you messages of un-ease. For me subliminal stress was caused by such mundane things as too-snug leg elastic on tight underwear, or pantyhose that were obviously too small. For others it may be an overfull belly, a binding waistband, or, for a woman, the lack of a well-supporting foundation garment. Understanding that all the events and objects in our life are wordlessly "talking" to us every moment of our lives can help us bring subliminal cues to awareness so that we can make conscious decisions to change them. You may be wearing too-snug clothes because you're ashamed to go shopping, though clothes that really fit without binding and straining might be a wonderful relief for your body, putting it out of its present misery.

Someone once spoke to me of the intractability of fat people's "deep-seated anxieties," but "deep-seated anxieties" are probably nothing more than garden-variety anxieties practiced with more passion and dedication than usual. On the other hand, as Chapter 6 mentioned, compulsive people are those who may feel emotional stress more keenly than others whenever they are careless about maintaining their own endorphins at a high level. Still, the biology-is-destiny question is much less compelling than the ability to find a tool or process that can foster serenity *now*.

Many people feel helpless in the face of negative emotions because they think such mental states happen *to* them. Everyone has negative moments, of course, but staying in them is a choice. Awareness can help clarify how that choice is made. If you found yourself feeling bored, for example, you might realize that you wouldn't need to be bored—alienated from your task—if you chose to focus with absorbed concentration on whatever you were doing. (The photographer Diane Arbus said, "The Chinese have a theory that you pass through boredom into fascination and I think it's true.") A classic anecdote illustrating this point is Gallwey's description of becoming fascinated by minute sights and sounds during an hour's freeway driving during the evening rush. He concluded that if he and his wife could be happy listening to freeway traffic, they would never have to fear boredom.

Awareness helped me become conscious of my individual eating cues. I discovered that I overate not only when I was feeling any of the standard negative emotions (boredom, anger, resentment, fear, etc.), but also when I felt abandoned; victimized (or the "abandoned victim"); isolated, uneasy, or unconfident; or ugly. These were once precise releasers of my compulsive behavior; in fact, anyone noticing me engaging in compulsive behavior could have reliably predicted that my mental state was one of the above. The triggering action was swift and severe in its effect, as the following anecdote shows. Once on a vacation we stopped at my in-laws' house for a few days. Our daughter was sick, so I stayed home to care for her while the rest of the family went out to dinner. The car had no sooner pulled out of the driveway than I found myself rushing to the freezer to gobble up most of a quart of ice cream. Later I wondered, pathetically, why I had jeopardized nearly a week's worth of sensible eating so suddenly and so senselessly, especially when I was supposed to be caring for a sick child? Much later I realized that I had subconsciously interpreted my being left alone in the house as abandonment, and I was simply pushed into my habitual response to that feeling.

The real obstacle to your weight loss may be only indirectly related to the food you put in your mouth, but much more closely connected to your frustrations about something else in your life (such as your husband, children, in-laws). That problem or problems may be what you *really* need to face before you can hope to get thin. And that's another truth it's best to face squarely: if presently your life is an appalling, tangled mess and you know you could never feel peaceful for a moment, for God's sake don't even think of losing weight right now. Put all your energies into cleaning up the muddle, and put off working on your weight problem until you are—at least in a relative sense—more serene.

As I mentioned in Chapter 9, Dorothy Tennov suggests that feeling the negative emotion as a body sensation may help pinpoint its cause. In *Being and Caring,* Daniels and Horowitz suggest noticing your body posture: "Pay special attention when you get into failure-talk inside your head. Notice the body position you go into when you feel like a failure. Exaggerate it.... From then on, whenever you notice that you're in your 'failure posture,' move into a posture that lets you feel good in your body." In fact, you can use the occurrence of the negative emotion itself, when you're aware, to remind you to substitute a better one, thus forging a new link in a conditioned response.

We need to release or discharge negative emotions and their associated bodily tensions before they get a grip on us and further influence our behavior. There are many ways: crying, laughing, talking it over with someone, vigorous exercise (see William Glasser's *Positive Addiction*), or journal writing (see either Ira Progoff's *At a Journal Workshop* or *Dr. Schiff's Miracle Weight-Loss Guide*). As Chapter 8 indicated, it also helps simply to hand the problem over to a higher authority for guidance and direction—anyone from a trusted, sympathet-

ic friend or doctor to a loving personal God. A group such as Weight
Watchers, TOPS, or Overeaters Anonymous can definitely provide
help with the struggle for serenity and personal growth. The nonjudg-
mental support of the group, the encouragement to share stressful
feelings, and a structured way of practicing good eating behavior may
provide just the help you need.

We call it *serenity* when the mind is free of tension; we call it *relaxation* when the body is. They are really one and the same; serenity
starts with the relaxation of the body. Maltz tells us that "it is absolutely impossible to feel fear, anger, anxiety, or negative emotions of
any kind while the muscles of the body are kept perfectly relaxed."
For a compulsive personality, relaxation may not come easy or naturally at first. Richard Hittleman says, "Simply observing that a muscle is tense is not enough in the beginning; *you must give it the order
to relax.*"

The daily practice of meditation is invaluable. Anyone who already
practices a specific meditation discipline, such as Transcendental
Meditation, at a specific time once or twice a day is very much ahead
of the game; those who don't should consider beginning. Read Benson's *The Relaxation Response* to discover that you don't need to pay
high fees or do anything difficult or esoteric to reap the enormous
benefits of regular relaxation training. Consult Kenneth Pelletier's
Mind as Healer, Mind as Slayer for a description of several meditative techniques that can induce deep relaxation. In *The Master Game*
Robert de Ropp says, "The first rule is very simple: *enter the silence
as often as possible; remain there for as long as possible.*"

Two fifteen- or twenty-minute sessions a day are enough to get going. Because we are so used to "doing," meditation may feel strange
because there's "nothing to do," though that's actually an illusion. As
you continue to practice meditation, you are making the pathway to
relaxation more and more assured, repeating and practicing behavior
that represents the antithesis of stress for both the body and the mind.
As *Twelve Steps and Twelve Traditions* points out, "Let's always remember that meditation is in reality intensely practical. One of its
first fruits is emotional balance."

But compulsive eaters (like smokers, alcoholics, drug addicts, etc.)
may be *more* anxiety-prone than the general population. We are those
who need to find a way to stay focused and calm and in our right
minds all during the day, not just for fifteen minutes morning and eve-

ing. At first, you may have to consciously stop your habitual anxious responses by substituting a command like "Calm." Though this may seem strange at first, as you practice, the once-unfamiliar behavior will become more and more automatic as the synapse in the brain is reinforced. A helpful tool is the use of a continuous meditative discipline to block out anxious thoughts, such as a soothing mantra (for example, "calm and grateful" said over and over all day long). If this sounds crazy to you, reread Salinger's *Franny,* with its description of the potent power of the Jesus Prayer, "prayed without ceasing." No matter what you call it—prayer, or mantra, or even constructive muttering—it's all the same on the physiological level.

When I get into situations that I know will get my Type A dander up (a traffic jam or a ridiculously long supermarket line, say), I automatically shift into being very absorbed in noticing and counting the intake and outgo of my breath. I do this until I can be serene on my own again. Consciously relaxing by means of this absorbed attention to something else actually blocks the stress response my body would normally be making, so it's biochemically true: I *can* cope better.

Timothy Gallwey says over and over in each of his books that, although he developed the concept of Inner Game to be used in sports, anyone can apply the concept to any "game" he happens to be playing. Dychtwald's *Body-Mind* defines meditative consciousness as the state in which "you are totally and selflessly involved in an activity to the point that there is little or no separation between you and what you are doing." Indeed, the notion of one's life as the truest meditative path is central to Zen practice. In *The Way of Everyday Life* Hakuyu Taizan Maezumi observes, "We shouldn't confuse this 'way' with some technique, or with some road for traveling someplace else. This way itself, this life itself, is realization. . . . To do very ordinary things in a very ordinary way—that's the buddha way."

The serenity we're talking about, then, is not a matter of actions so much as an ongoing state of mind. In order to keep the spirit of serenity operating in your life, you may need to be willing to do a little less, since overbusy "doing" leads to the Type A "hurry sickness" and a consequent neglect of the smaller details of what you are doing. If you're trying to lose weight meditatively, you need to choose a period of time that you want to savor—one that you wouldn't *want* to be over with any more quickly than it is (for instance, summer). Then you set about your "doing" in a spirit of savoring the present moment, keeping yourself focused on the details of the effort to the exclusion of anxious self-consciousness. The Lamaze method uses relaxation and concentrated focus to make the stress of childbirth bearable without resort to anesthesia or drugs. Think of my recommendations as Lamaze for dieters.

This approach has many related benefits in other areas of your life. I was once told by a YMCA swimming instructor that I was so tense she didn't see how I made it across the pool at all; being able to relax at will has immeasurably helped my ability to swim. I recently took a course in voice improvement from Dr. Morton Cooper, the noted voice specialist. Most of his work with individual class members was nothing more than undoing the laryngal tension that was preventing them from projecting their resonant natural voice.

Another thing that helps is to realize that you are only as much as the feelings you are expressing at any given moment. Try to bring into your life as much reason to feel joyful as you can. If necessary, recall past experiences of joy and embroider them in your mind—dwelling upon them, recreating them. As you give yourself up more and more to feeling ongoing joy, you will find to your immense astonishment and relief that the burden of your anxious self-consciousness and self criticism is being lifted from you.

It is equally important to understand that all the pursuits you undertake for personal satisfaction are fundamentally a search not for the experience itself, the "doing," but for the pleasant state of mind associated with that experience. The physical act of sex is less significant than the *feeling* of being desired and cherished, and sex problems result when the feelings are missing. I used to love eating out (or rather, *overeating* out) in restaurants. Then I realized that what I really liked about going to restaurants was the agreeable feeling of being all dressed up, feeling "special," feeling festive, and so on. Once I saw that it was the *feelings* that gave me the greatest pleasure, I could become less obsessed with the food I was eating. In fact, I even came to understand that ordering only a salad and a glass of iced tea did nothing to diminish my pleasure in dining out, and that all the extra food I used to eat was just a misguided definition of satisfaction.

To state it as simply as possible: it's important always to attempt to meet your needs in the way they should be met. That sounds easy, but for chronic overeaters it's not. Meeting your needs means to look for and obtain your due rewards in life. Not only are we reluctant to claim all our due rewards, but we've also been misguidedly rewarding ourselves with food, a "reward" that is really a punishment. All addictions are just substitutes for more genuine human pleasures. Everyone has the right to a certain amount of satisfaction out of life; overeaters do too, but they've been trained to look for a disproportionate amount of their life's satisfaction in food.

Overeaters habitually use food as the avenue to a different state of mind—as Anne Scott Beller remarks, "Food is the cheapest and most abundant mood-altering drug on the market." But the trip doesn't last. The constant repetitive search for satisfaction from food brings to mind Hans Christian Andersen's pathetic little match girl, constantly striking bundles of matches to momentarily transport herself into dream realms where she wasn't tired, hungry, and cold. But the blaze of the matches—intoxicating while it lasts—always fades. Overeating is like that. exciting, illusory, and ultimately lethal. We need to start searching for more genuine rewards that will bring more genuine, lasting satisfaction. A man who had once been fat told me he had finally become able to ask for and search out what he really needs—affection—rather than settling for the solitary pleasures of overeating.

This chapter will close with an additional word about mantras. Most people connect the use of mantras with meditation, though a few pages ago I mentioned using a mantra all day long to help foster ongoing serenity. It's important to understand how mantras work. They aren't just mumbo-jumbo; they have a definite, measurable effect on the operation of the brain. The use of a Sanskrit or nonsense syllable for a mantra can alter consciousness simply by boring to death (and therefore turning off) the word-processing left hemisphere of the brain so that the right hemisphere can dominate. Right-hemisphere dominance is associated with higher levels of alpha waves, that is, a more relaxed state. But a mantra doesn't have to be a nonsense syllable; it can be a short phrase that conveys the essence of a desired goal. The constant repetition of such a phrase can serve as a constant subliminal reinforcement of your goal. The next chapter will discuss in greater detail how to phrase your desired goals so that the bodymind can recognize them and begin making them into reality.

12
Setting Inner Goals

Chiang spoke slowly.... "To fly as fast as thought, to anywhere that is," he said, "you must begin by knowing that you have already arrived."
Richard Bach, *Jonathan Livingston Seagull*

Ridding yourself of unconscious pervasive anxiety will do more than anything else to set you on the right road toward shedding that "excess" weight you no longer want. But calmness is only one half of the game your mind can play; the other half is to fill your life with positive experiences and visualizations—real and imagined beneficial feedback—so that being more attractive is a natural outcome.

It has long been conventional medical wisdom that a woman is as close to her ideal weight as she will ever be on her wedding day, though doctors never bothered to ask why this should be so. The answer is clear. A bride-to-be receives constant praise and good feedback not only from her fiance, but also from the rest of her circle of acquaintances, who are temporarily turned into her adoring courtiers. Her bodymind has no choice but to act on all these unanimous instructions and make her into someone as perfect as it is possible for her to be. (Later in this chapter I will discuss why for some brides this perfection is a size 8 and for others a size 18.)

Back when I believed that falling in love had some magical restorative cosmetic powers, I was married and fat. I thought to myself, "How inconvenient! I'm happily married and I don't want to have to take a lover just to get thin." But not long after that I discovered that *all* pleasant, nonstressful, absorbing experiences contained a common factor capable of bringing about desired personal changes. When I could see that, I was nearly ready to understand that each of us can supply our own good feedback instead of waiting for the outside world to provide it for us.

I was still struggling with the problem of thinking of myself as impossibly ugly and was unable to redefine myself any other way when I came across this phrase in Fred Rohé's *The Zen of Running:* "We create the quality of our own experience." It was like a thunderbolt. I suddenly saw that I was choosing to perceive *only* those experiences that convinced me I was fat and worthless (and was choosing to interpret all my experiences as further evidence of it). As I mentioned earlier, I have always lived close to the beach, but I almost never went there. My implicit thought was, "You're too ugly to deserve to go to the beach like all those beautiful-bodied people. You don't belong there." Nonsense! I suddenly saw that the game itself was neutral; I could choose to play it as any kind of player I wanted to be.

Next I looked into my closet and was appalled by what I found there. With my new awareness I saw all too clearly that my clothes reflected with devastating accuracy my low self-image. The clothes were not cheap ones, but they seemed to have been deliberately selected to minimize the wearer's attractiveness. This was what I had always called "my taste"—timid color and cut, boring shapes. I consciously rejected clothes that seemed too adventurous (read fashionable) for "my taste." Then I realized what an idiotic straitjacket I had been putting myself into; my clothes were constant subliminal reinforcements to me, continually strengthening my tendency to be an unattractive, unsexy woman. I went right out and bought all new lacy underwear (which never had seemed "me" before); I went on a modest shopping spree for a few items, like soft crepe blouses I had never worn before (not "practical" enough). I marched into my sewing room and began to put together an entirely new kind of wardrobe, whose textures and fabrics were completely different from anything I had formerly worn. By the next month I had worked up to seeing myself in (and therefore buying myself) wonderful lacy nightgowns—as unlike the previous "me" as anyone could imagine. My husband was delighted.

If you identify with my story so far and think a similar revelation would help you, read on. The rest of the chapter presents the principles that informed these experiences, which are applicable to both men and women. It isn't necessary for your life to be exactly like mine for you to gain an understanding of how to set your own inner goals and go about pursuing them in a spirit of joy, inner peacefulness, and not-trying.

What Fred Rohé says is true in the most basic, most literal sense: each of us indeed creates the quality of our own experience. Each of us sets and attains goals as well as we know how. But as members of this particular culture we are severely handicapped in our attempts, since our culture's general view of how to solve problems—direct attack— has almost nothing to do with the reality of how our bodyminds go about reaching the goals we set for ourselves in our personal lives. As pragmatists, we're always much more interested in ends than in means, but for personal development or accomplishment the "means whereby" is *all there is*. Therefore, when we talk about a goal as if it were a thing, we are really understanding only its *name,* not its sub- stance; we must understand that any goal is a *process* before we can begin to grasp how to start getting there.

Contrary to what seems intuitively true, the conscious, "talking" part of our mind does very little toward achieving our goals; the cre- ative, goal-seeking mechanism is the subconscious mind, or bodymind. The conscious mind knows only how to manipulate words and plays the role of commentator. The talking self understands only the name of the goal (getting thin), not the goal itself (the experiences required to bring it about). The conscious and unconscious parts of the mind seem to speak different languages. The problem is that we listen atten- tively to the talking self, while we barely know how to contact, let alone communicate with, the subconscious mind. The conscious mind, or left hemisphere of the brain, represents the way we have been taught to use and interpret language since infancy, but the subcon- scious mind's semantic understanding is very different (in fact, some- times nearly backward) from that.

For a moment let's think of our goal as a tangible process—build- ing a house, let's say. If you cared at all about what your house would look like when it was finished, you'd be very careful about supplying clear instructions to the builder and having on hand the best possible raw materials. The absence of either would be detrimental in the long run. Words and how they are used are the essence of the clear instruc- tions. Keep in mind that your builder's native tongue is not the same as your own, which makes it necessary to be extremely careful in what you say to ensure that accurate communication takes place. We are suggestible creatures, and words can influence our bodyminds; that's why we have to be careful to discipline what we say to ourselves. Our talking mind is like the apprentice bricklayer: if trained, he can be helpful; if wayward, he knocks over all the bricks and hinders progress all around.

Here are the essential pitfalls of communicating with our subconscious mind, as they were explained to me by Susan Newton. The subconscious mind doesn't understand anything but now (the future is an endless succession of "nows"). It can't grasp anything phrased in the negative, because it understands only how to "do" something, not how to "not do" something. As Chapter 7 explained, when you say "should," the subconscious mind understands that as "I don't want to." Can you see the difficulty? When we give ourselves our twice-weekly self-improvement lecture, most of us talk like this: "I should lose some weight. I'd like to be thin by next week, because I'm so fat and ugly now." To the subconscious mind, "I should lose some weight" is understood as "I don't want to lose some weight." The phrase "I'd like to be thin next week" means "I'm not thin today," and since, to the subconscious, time is only an infinite series of "todays," thin will never arrive. "I'm so fat and ugly" means that's my vision of myself—the goal I'm pursuing.

When you phrase your "goals" in this negative way, your subconscious mind has no choice but to misunderstand you; it will continue to provide you with fatness and self-dissatisfaction until you learn to speak its language and tell it that this was not what you had in mind. The essence of incorrect mental programming is the pursuit of negative goals. Because the subconscious mind can't understand the negative, when "not being fat" is your goal, it will be forever unattainable. Your goal has to be "getting thinner," and you must *feel* what it would be like to attain your goal even before you arrive. In *Mind Over Platter,* Dr. Peter Lindner observed, "The subconscious mind has proved time and again that it can make no error if it is programmed correctly.... You must visualize yourself exactly as you wish to be. This means you must 'see' your body as it should be and recognize the program that will result in this goal." He adds, "It is important that you produce a feeling of euphoria as you contemplate your new image." Maltz expands upon this idea with the following observation: "When we set out to find a new idea, or the answer to a problem, *we must assume that the answer exists already—somewhere,* and set out to find it. Dr. Norbert Wiener has said, 'Once a scientist attacks a

problem which he knows to have an answer, his entire attitude i
changed. He is already some fifty percent of his way toward that an
swer.'"

To return to our analogy with house building, it is visualized expe
riences such as these that are the raw materials for the construction
You have to project how it would *feel* to be happy with your body.
then *practice* feeling those feelings over and over, until the outcome is
inevitable. You may find it difficult to engender feelings of euphoria
about yourself if all you've ever practiced is self-criticism. You emphatically won't be able to think any better of yourself than you presently do if you won't permit yourself to have experiences that prove to
you you're a worthy person, or a person who can reach the goals
you've set. As Maltz tells us, "Our present state of self-confidence and
poise is the result of what we have 'experienced' rather than what we
have learned intellectually."

George Masters' book about his beauty secrets contains this memorable description of what happened to women after they had had the
Masters treatment: "They come to life. When they *look* good, they
feel good. Their personalities change in a minute. It's like a butterfly
emerging from a cocoon. They have more oomph, self-confidence, the
instant ability to *project* something they never had before. . . . There is
an indisputable transformation in a woman—any woman—when the
feeling of being beautiful takes over."

Feeling ugly is something you *choose,* and when you choose it, you
are in fact pursuing it as a goal. We choose every moment of our lives
if you keep choosing the experiences you've always had, it goes without saying that you'll keep the body you've always had, too. It is a vicious circle: feeling unattractive, we simply cannot feel worthy of all
the nice experiences we see thin people having (such as my never allowing myself to go to the beach). As we sit on the sidelines, not par-
ticipating, we inevitably lock ourselves into further self-consciousness
and self-obsession about overweight. But if we never let ourselves have
any nice experiences, we're making it much more difficult to visualize
anything other than what we have.

A friend once told me that her food binging and her sex life were
reciprocal in a very direct sense; when she wasn't feeling sexually satisfied, she felt herself turning (mentally) into less of a woman and
more of a child, with a correspondingly greater need for the childish
comfort of food. On the other hand, when her sexual needs were being

met, she didn't think about binging at all. As noted brain physiologist Karl Pribram observed in a UCLA lecture, "When you're hungry you're not sexy; when you're sexy you're not hungry."

The ugly witch and the princess of the fairy tales are not two discrete characters, but a continuum. We can locate ourselves at whatever point we choose along that continuum. Since in our culture we tend to be thing-oriented rather than process-oriented, it is hard for us to see that every living being is indeed a process. Your ideal body is in fact *here now;* you are living in it, underneath your fat. Most people see "getting thin" almost as becoming another person—as if one were a character in a book and had to become another character instead. When you do get thin, you will have made some fairly important personal changes, but they are all part of the process that is you. You don't have to switch identities to be thin: you are a thin person already, inside your fat person.

In the first chapter I introduced the notion of the thin mind-set, that prior set of self-convictions around which our actions organize themselves. There are always at least two ways to look at every experience in your life; you probably have more practice in the anxious, self-critical interpretation than in the relaxed and self-accepting one. Remember the discussion in Chapter 9 about the well-worn diet book advice to go out and buy yourself a too-small dress to be your "motivation." You can, like most people, choose to feel threatened by this; seeing the small dress and knowing you can't get into it can make you feel anxious and depressed. But there is a more serene approach to the same problem. Instead of buying the dress (and immediately fretting that you're too big to fit into it), substitute meditative experiences in which you visualize yourself looking marvelous in the dress. Don't focus on the "not" of the experiences, but construct some reassuring, enlivening components of it. There's a big difference between my telling myself, "You're so ugly—you can't possibly go to the beach until you take off some of that flab," and saying instead, "Nancy, you have the makings of a terrific tap dancer (soccer player, swimmer, runner). Why don't you lose a little weight?"

Everything is a function of context. There may not be a woman alive in this country today who likes the shape of her thighs, yet we have all had the experience of gazing at a hefty ancient or modern statue of a woman and feeling swept away on a tide of compelling femaleness. Does Lachaise's monumental *Standing Woman* in the courtyard of New York's Museum of Modern Art look like the type of woman who spends any time at all worrying about those thighs of hers? Not a chance. In other words, you have to understand that you're a terrific-looking big person before you can entertain any hopes of becoming a terrific-looking small person. If you're a woman who doesn't even know where to begin in feeling better about yourself, get a copy of Stella Reichman's *Great Big Beautiful Doll*. A man can read Laurence Reich's *From Fat to Skinny*. It will be the start of a new life.

Timothy Gallwey's Inner Game books describe all the mental enemies of such serenity—the "uh-oh" experience, the "ho hums," and so forth. The game of becoming thin has an equal number of mental pitfalls, of which the following are only a small selection.

Measuring oneself against a standard of perfection. This apparently laudable pursuit of quality is nothing but an invitation to dissatisfaction and self-hatred. Unfortunately, advertising relentlessly tries to make us uneasy by constantly projecting images of physical perfection, unrealistically ectomorphic to boot. But advertising is static; people are processes. The definition of truly being alive is to be *moving toward* perfection. We would be much better off, therefore, if we would simply ignore the perfection we see in advertising in favor of absorption in our own growth process.

Daydreaming. I can just hear someone objecting, "I'm convinced that programming the subconscious mind doesn't work the way you say it does because I fantasize being thin all the time and I'm still not." Fantasizing and daydreaming may be a start, but when they don't get you where you want to go, it's because they aren't focused enough, intent enough, detailed enough. A daydream is a very vague "I wish I were" kind of mental noodling; programming the subconscious mind is a discipline, an ability to stay focused on the goal, feeling strongly the emotions associated with the desired state.

"Tomorrow" psychology. Fat people have certain self-defeating notions about not being "deserving" of good things because of being fat. I used to talk like this: I can't buy new clothes until I'm thin; I can't join an exercise class until I look better in a leotard; I'll never get a new boyfriend (husband, whatever) until I'm not fat any more. All of these are stupid choices that leave you in a continuing limbo of "not-yet," having antiexperiences. I spent more than thirty years in the land of not-yet, and I can't tell you how good it felt to move to the new neighborhood of "right now."

Many of us have already decided that losing weight is an unpleasant process (which my own experiences, for one, refute). Because we have defined discipline negatively, we are prepared for unpleasant rigor and self-mortification. But there is no natural motivation to continue unpleasant experiences. When we *do* discontinue them, our talking self criticizes us once more for lacking will power, when the real problem was insufficient imagination: finding a *pleasant* means to the same end.

Fred Rohé sums up the issue very well by saying, "It's your choice of whether you run to *punish* your self or to *experience* your self." Any experience has two components: the ostensible and the subliminal. The ostensible component of calisthenics, for example, is nothing but agreeable: how good for you it is, how healthy, and so on. But the subliminal component of calisthenics (how you *actually* experience it, as opposed to how you are *supposed* to be experiencing it) is boredom to the *n*th degree. You can't pursue the desirable goal without resenting the bad side effects. If getting physically fit is the goal, look for a way to do it that really *is* fun: Aerobic Dancing®, Jazzercise®, disco dancing, tap dancing, whatever. Don't waste your time doing anything you're not really enthralled with.

If you aren't liking what you're doing, the problem may be that you don't have a large enough sense of the meaning of your goal—what you're doing it for. Here's an example of my own. Having decided to get more physically fit through running, I found I didn't care too much for running in and of itself. When I joined a women's soccer team, however, I perceived the need for that training very differently than I had before. When running was the ultimate goal, it seemed boring, but when it helped me achieve *another* important goal, I did it willingly. Before I played soccer, I told myself not only that I didn't like running but also that, if I did run, a mile was the absolute limit I could ever endure. One day, feeling particularly fine, I decided on the spur of the moment to run two miles instead of one. To my amazement, the second mile was nearly effortless—only imperceptibly more taxing than running the first. Without making some effort to find out if my self-imposed judgment was real or not, I could have been stuck in a silly, limiting self-concept that didn't even fit the facts!

It isn't what you do so much as how you do it. The *what* you do is only the name of the goal; the *how* you do it is the essence of the process itself. The metagoal beyond your immediate goal is to keep the right spirit intact as you go. An analogy with courtship can help explain how to acquire patience and willingness, the two most important mental states for goal-striving success. Losing weight ought to feel like being engaged; the desired goal may be a long way off, but getting there ought to be so delightful that impatience would be pointless.

Willingness transforms any endeavor; in fact, it is willingness, rather than available knowledge or resources, that primarily determines success. Consider the following two scenarios. In the first you are being asked to cook dinner for some disagreeable people. You unwillingly shuffle through your cookbooks (your knowledge of "what to do"), not finding anything satisfactory. The meal is a disaster. In the second scenario you are cooking for your lover. You enthusiastically riffle through the *same* cookbooks, read the *same* recipes (dieting methods), but now ideas nearly pop out of the pages at you; you cook a creative, innovative meal and it's a smashing success.

Lack of success may be the result of phrasing your goals so that their significance is not conveyed to the bodymind. You need to understand and express the larger *idea* before the "how to do it" will become apparent in your life. Here are two other ways of phrasing this idea. Instead of "trying to get thin," arrange your life so that overeating is not necessary in it, and choose a larger life goal that is incompatible with remaining fat.

As I have observed before, it is difficult for doers such as ourselves to accept the idea that anything as passive as visualizing a result could make it happen (though our gullibility leads us to accept the magic in diet pills without a qualm). Sometimes all the happy, serene visualizations in the world don't bring about any measurable change. Why? Why are some "perfect" brides not as thin as others? What limits their ability to reach ultimate, not just relative, thinness?

The first important criterion is the intensity of your concentration, for this is what makes the difference between vagueness and specificity. As Maltz says, "You must have a clear mental picture of the correct thing before you can do it successfully." Later he writes, "*Details* of the imagined environment are all-important in this exercise, because for all practical purposes, you are creating a *practice experience.* . . . Experimental and clinical psychologists have proved beyond a shadow of a doubt that the human nervous system cannot tell the difference between an 'actual' experience and an experience *imagined vividly and in detail.*" Paul Hawken's beautiful book *The Magic of Findhorn* contains this sentence: "You are what you think, you become what you think, and what you think becomes reality."

Brain physiologists seem to be on the verge of a startling validation of this idea. Brain nerve endings have been observed to generate interference patterns, the raw material of holograms, those strange three-dimensional pictures that look real. Your concentrated goal-seeking thoughts, practiced enough, may create in your mind a neurological filter, so to speak, that fosters the realization of your chosen reality by a sort of anticipation or matching process. As one textbook on brain function, Tyler and Dawson's *Current Neurology,* explained, "These mechanisms all mean that the brain is not a passive recipient of external sensation, but that much if not all of the time it has already constructed an anticipatory internal representation of what it expects to find. In this respect, most activities become an act of recognition and of matching an external input or output to an inner replica."

When you use a projector, you need to bring the picture into clear focus before you can see anything. The image is there, registered on the film, but it makes no sense to the viewer until it is focused properly. I found when writing this book that just wanting to write it was ludicrously inadequate; I had to focus my intention very clearly by means of extremely detailed chapter outlines before I could put any of the chapters onto paper.

Prayer is another name for achieving goals, and it has a cybernetic component as well. In *A Gift of Wings,* Richard Bach says, "Whatever we wrap away in thought is opened for us, one day, in experience. . . . The world is as it is because that is the way we wish it to be. Only as our wish changes does the world change. Whatever we pray for, we get." Sometimes your request may be granted immediately; sometimes all you are given is a pointer to the path which leads to the learning that must be mastered before the goal is reached. In fact, some of the learning you are required to do may involve less than pleasant experiences. But, given the hologram theory of the brain, you hold in your mind the picture of your future. While you do the "footwork," your imagination will help bring what you want into being. When you find yourself resistant and unwilling to be disciplined in a manner that leads to the goal, this is only a sign that you do not fully perceive yourself as fitting into the universe in which that particular goal resides.

The subconscious mind not only looks at the visualizations you give it, but it also implicitly asks the question, "What is this for?" It needs to know the meaning of what you're trying to do: why do you want it? If you can't specify that, then you have only incompletely specified the goal. Once again, Timothy Gallwey provides an eloquent explanation of how to see your goals as fully as possible:

As I acquire an increased sense of my overall purpose as a human being, it in turn becomes easier to answer the question of what I really want in day-to-day situations. And the better I see the connection between my overall purpose and my daily activities, the greater the sense of meaning and the higher the level of interest I will develop. Thus, knowing what you want is a constant process of paying attention to your experiences, both internal and external, and of refining your sense of purpose.

You may be very accomplished at seeing yourself in a size 8 bikini, but if your image is essentially a paper doll—like a still photo instead of a movie—your imagination may still be insufficient to communicate its specifications to the bodymind. If you can vividly visualize the *entire process*, the whole universe, of your thinness (the way you would be eating, the exercise you'd be getting), then you are virtually guaranteed success.

The best context, of course, is a continuous feeling of euphoria. Euphoria is a natural result of feeling attractive and desirable, so practice feeling that way (and don't be discouraged if it doesn't come easy at the beginning). Gallwey explains how to get over beginner's problems, no matter what it is you're doing: "I pick a quality in which I believe I am lacking, one which I think doesn't usually manifest itself. Then I focus on it, however little of it there seems to be, and try to express it in my play." To reliably create ongoing euphoria, you may need a continuous goal-reminding mantra that you say to yourself all day long; don't feel self-conscious about using one, since no one but you knows you're doing it. It's the surest way to stay focused and intent upon what you want to accomplish. For several months I used "thin and sexy"; maybe you will come up with a better one. As soon as you begin losing some weight, you won't have to *try* to create the euphoria any longer, for you will get into that natural high which comes with feeling healthier and more energetic, wearing attractive new clothes, being complimented by those around you, and so on.

Remember my remarks in Chapter 11 about your constant subliminal dialogue with your environment. Arrange as many details of your surroundings as possible so that they reflect back to all your senses an ideal world. Play gratifying music all day—music that makes you feel happy, or sexy. (One of the girls in my college dorm used to play

Ravel's *Bolero* before every date. I thought she was crazy, but now I'm pretty sure she was on the right track.) If you're a woman, buy yourself flowers; no one deserves them more than you. If you're a man, indulge yourself with other gifts. Raysa Rose Bonow's fine book *How to Be a Thin Person* constantly repeats, "Be kind to yourself." Yes: be as kind to yourself as you possibly can. In *From Fat to Skinny,* Dr. Laurence Reich tells a poignant anecdote of needless self-denial about a woman who could never bring herself to wear perfume when she was fat:

"There was no rhyme or reason to it," she said. "I just associated perfume with slender, sexy women. It seemed ridiculous for me at my weight to use the stuff. When I decided I was going to knock off my extra weight, I went out and bought a small bottle of perfume. . . . Then came the day when I lost the weight I planned to. What a thrill it was to use that perfume!"

Wear your perfume *now!* Your five senses compose your inner view of what kind of a person you are, and they can't work for you unless you are willing to provide a little help.

An overweight unmarried man is likely to deny himself the pleasure of asking women out on dates, both from a feeling of worthlessness and a fear of being rejected. A very subtle, and self-fulfilling, loser's strategy is to become careless about one's personal hygiene and the cleanliness of one's living quarters. The subconscious thought "It's OK for the place to look like this, because no woman is likely to ever come here anyway" is the best possible insurance that any woman who did come for a visit would be less than beguiled by the experience.

Before you lose any weight, buy yourself at least one great-looking outfit to wear when you are tempted to feel doubtful about yourself again. Make sure your outfit fits you well, and completely ignore that little voice inside you that keeps advising, "Don't spend a lot of money on this—you won't be able to wear it any more when you get thin." Any diet aid (and clothes fall into that category) is by definition something you won't need once you're thin—but it makes all the difference in the world right now.

Go through your wardrobe and minutely analyze every garment you regularly wear in order to discover unknown uncomfortablenesses that engender negative body messages. If you are a woman, see if your dresses fit well without binding or ballooning, if your pantyhose feel ample and stretchy. If you are a man, check the fit of slacks, shirts, and underwear. If your clothes are too tight, buy yourself larger sizes without hating yourself for it. I started wearing Big Mama pantyhose when I was fat because I needed more room, but I still wear them now that I'm thinner, because they just feel agreeably ample. For further positive messages to yourself, make sure that your clothes and underthings are clean and well-cared-for (remember, Joan Didion wasn't *recommending* safety pins in people's underwear).

Here is a brief list of pleasure-enhancing tools that can help you make your goals a reality. If there's any item you don't have or use regularly, ask yourself searchingly whether it's because you've never thought you were worthy of it. For women: pretty clothes, perfume, cosmetics and eye makeup, a silky-feeling body lotion, flowers, pretty lingerie and nightwear, good-looking dishes and glassware, and books on grooming and personal attractiveness. For men: well-cut suits and other clothes, carefully chosen accessories, a becoming haircut, personal toiletries (including cologne), acceptably clean living quarters, attractive dishes and glassware, and grooming books. Then use them to construct a personal universe that is so satisfying to you that you can't *help* being happy with yourself. When you're feeling that way, and expressing that feeling out in the world, you infinitely magnify your chances of attracting other nice people into your world to share your happiness with you.

13
Messages from Your Body, 2: Balance and Imbalance

"Forget about faith!" Chiang said it time and again.
"You didn't need faith to fly, you needed to understand
flying."
Richard Bach, *Jonathan Livingston Seagull*

Earlier in this book I complained that most other diet books were very long on information but short on wisdom. I claimed that lifelong readers of diet books already have much more knowledge about the subject than they need. This chapter may seem as though I'm contradicting myself, providing more of that boring and intimidating information that can't be used effectively in one's personal life. But everything in this chapter is a fact or an insight that once came as a surprise to me even when I thought I already knew a great deal. Each was like a missing piece of a puzzle in helping me organize my knowledge better; each helped explain my body to me and helped us become better friends. All the facts that dieters know about dieting are like beads dropped on the floor: useless until strung together. This chapter takes the all-too-familiar "facts" about losing weight and assembles them into a coherent structure to help you gain insight into the meaning of your weight-loss (or weight-gain) experiences. The aim is not only to supply more information, but to show you what your knowledge *means*; it will make it possible for you to live amicably with your body and to accept what it must do to keep you alive and healthy.

When I drive my car, I am aware that I do not make the car go; that is the engine's job. I am there only to do the steering. It is useful to me to know as much as I can about how the motor works, because that will help keep me out of trouble with the car. But all my knowledge about the workings of the motor should not give me the erroneous impression that I am the one responsible for supplying power to the car. The same is true of our bodies and the temptation of our conscious minds to take control, believing that they know best how to "make it go."

Let's get back for a moment to the question of how we put together the body of knowledge we call "what we know." Some approaches to overweight seem to view what is basically a physiological issue with a moralizing, jaundiced eye. Needless to say, these cannot help. In addition, many items of "gospel truth" about fatness are old wives' tales. We need to distinguish the bad information from the good, since only the genuine will provide useful feedback. Some of the wrong things you know may be ideas you cherish, but if they don't square with the facts, you're better off without them. Great awareness and sophistication are needed to pick and choose among all the available knowledge (and sometimes contradictory pronouncements) in this particular field.

Throughout this book I have stressed the need to rediscover *yourself* as your ultimate authority in questions of health. As always, we must begin with the notion of equilibrium, since everything about losing weight centers upon that. Remember the apparent paradox about your body: first, its equilibrium is not very healthy; second, you must listen to the messages it sends you as feedback. Clearly, if you are forced to listen to a body that isn't completely healthy, you will have to learn to distinguish between messages of disease and messages of health. This chapter will describe how diets tend to elicit the former; Chapter 14 will explain how to encourage more of the latter. Chapter 6 described the overall deranged and unstable condition that is caused by stress and in turn causes addictive behavior; this chapter will focus on the way we put ourselves temporarily out of balance through a misguided choice of diet.

We need to take a moment to look at some of our habituated cultural assumptions about food, both because our present patterns may sooner or later become obsolete owing to the pressures of a growing world population, and because (entirely independent of that) our present choices are lethal to us in the long run. Adams and Murray refer to "the fatal All-American-Supermarket-Madison-Avenue-TV-Ad-Teen-Age Diet, which is the diet of the average American." No matter how conscientious we think we usually are, these are the eating habits we rely on when we're overly rushed, which happens more than we like to admit: snacks at the local fast food outlet or frozen entrees from the supermarket. But, as Dr. George Watson wryly observes, "One simply can't take a 'day off' from sound nutrition."

Whenever we have anything to do with food that is "marketed"—brought to our attention via loud, expensive advertising campaigns—we are implicitly condoning an underlying assumption: that the point of food is *entertainment*. But the point of food is *not* entertainment; it is cell nourishment. However, if all of us—producers and consumers alike—see nothing wrong with the former view, then it is not in the least surprising that all the earnest attempts to improve our national eating habits are doomed to fail. If we believe that food is most fundamentally a "marketable commodity," we have made a serious error. Until now we have passively agreed to let ourselves be fed with food that has been altered until it no longer serves our cells' purposes very well. The late Dr. Thomas D. Spies is quoted in Cheraskin et al.'s *Diet and Disease:* "Our chief medical adversary is what I consider a disturbance of the inner balance of the constituents of our tissues, which are built from and maintained by the necessary chemicals in the air we breathe, the water we drink, and the food we eat." The high concentrations of salt and sugar in most processed food probably cannot be handled by the body without eliciting the stress response. Dr. John Yudkin points out in *Sweet and Dangerous* that, in our culture at least, we cannot use our instincts without caution:

Animals choose diets that they find palatable, but whatever these diets are, they must supply all their nutritional needs. If they did not, the animals would perish. . . . Many people still believe that foods that are palatable must *ipso facto* also have a high nutritional value. . . . I am certain that it is the dissociation of palatability and nutritional value that is the major cause of the "malnutrition of affluence."

Even more alarming, of course, is the way in which our toxic inner environment adversely affects our intestinal flora, the source of much of our energy-producing ability. The "good" bacteria in our intestines, lactobacillus acidophilus, grow best in slightly alkaline surroundings; the strong acidity associated with the presence of concentrated sugar encourages the growth of less desirable microorganisms as well. Virtuously, we consume yogurt, though our yogurt is so highly sweetened that its value may be questionable.

Interestingly enough, people with metabolic difficulties become habituated to them and then think of them as "business as usual." In *The Resurrection of the Body,* F. Matthias Alexander tells an affecting anecdote of straightening out the twisted body of a badly deformed girl, only to have her cry out, "Oh! Mummie, he's pulled me *out of shape."* Alexander comments, "When people are wrong, the thing which is right is bound to be wrong to them." People whose deranged metabolism is caused by persistent stress find it impossible to see their problem—or rather, they see *only* "problems" (tiredness, moodiness, and so forth) without being able to see the overall context in which the problems flourish. Dr. Grant Gwinup's comment (in Chapter 4) about people refusing to stay on an unbalanced diet for more than about three days referred to *normal* people. Addicts are people whose unbalanced need for the addictive substance has reached a point of tolerance where they don't "bounce back"; the addicted state "feels right." Null and Null's *Alcohol and Nutrition* reports one study in which "it was found that the appetite mechanism of malnourished children had become disturbed. When given a choice, the children would eat nothing but sugar in spite of an obvious need for other substances."

There are many kinds of fat people; in fact, they form a continuum ranging from those who were "always" overweight (that is, from fairly early in life onward) to those who once were of normal weight (perhaps most of their lives) until the slowing down of metabolism with advancing age or maybe pregnancy-induced carbohydrate intolerance changed their metabolic makeup. This metabolic continuum accounts for the wide variety of individualized reactions to standardized diets; it is why we need to fit the diet to the person, not vice versa. Much of the rest of this chapter will concern individual *symptoms,* each of which is not only related to the others but also an inevitable outcome given a body in unstable equilibrium (because of stress) or metabolic weakness (because of lack of digestive fitness).

All human bodies have two major metabolic pathways, the *ergotropic* (work-performing) and the *trophotropic* (food-storing). The former burns up calories doing work, the second stores them as fat. A body can become accustomed to using the latter pathway far more frequently than its owner would prefer. As Dr. Lawrence E. Lamb points out in *Metabolics,* "By forming fat a cell can process food we eat without requiring a lot of oxygen we normally need to release energy. This may be a very important factor in explaining why some overweight people always feel tired. Their cells use the 'no oxygen' processing route (fat path) to form fat rather than the 'high oxygen' route to release energy (energy circle)." However, as I will discuss later, the body can be coaxed and reeducated into greater use of the energy-burning pathway; Lamb comments, "Exercise increases circulation and oxygen delivery. At the same time it requires energy. One possible benefit from exercise may be to stimulate our cells to use the energy-releasing circle rather than the energy-storing fat path."

As long as we think of obese people as shameful gluttons, we are blind to the truth about them: far from being overnourished, most obese people suffer from subclinical malnutrition. Dr. H. L. Newbold says quite bluntly, "I consider obesity only another symptom of improper nutrition, like pellagra or scurvy." Those who have been obese all their lives suffer from the most severe forms of it; they are people whose cells are so inefficient at using the nutrients in food that overeating is inevitable for them, since their cells are constantly starved for the proper amounts and balance of nutrients that their faulty digestion cannot obtain properly from their food. Anyone who read Dr. Neil Solomon's book *The Truth About Weight Control* will probably remember his shocking statistics about metabolic abnormalities in the obese: 37 percent do not metabolize glucose properly; 73 percent have abnormal fat metabolism and 28 percent abnormal protein metabolism. Patients at the Lindner Clinic were told that obese people had up to twenty-six separate metabolic abnormalities, and that only reducing to normal weight could cure these. Such facts would be overwhelmingly pessimistic if it weren't for the fact that each of us, as an ongoing process, can decide to change any path we're on; according to Kenneth Pelletier, "A disorder is not a static manifestation of pathology, but rather a dynamic, developmental process. Any dynamic system can be altered away from pathology toward health, and that is a source of great optimism."

Part of the reason so many people feel helpless about being able to reduce to normal weight forever is that the first step has never been properly explained. It's a lot like going down the basement stairs in the dark when someone has kicked out the first step—you trip and fall all the way to the bottom. Going on a diet to get thin for good involves changing the body over from one equilibrium (the fat one) to another (the thin one). Given the inertia factor of our bodies (the required three-week changeover period mentioned in Chapter 3), an enormous amount of energy must be committed to the switch-over. Have you ever seen an ant trying to climb out of a glass bowl? It tries and tries, but can't muster up enough energy to get over the top. Getting thin takes that kind of energy at first, though ironically what you are supposed to do on a diet is to *reduce* your calories (and thus your available energy)!

No one in his right mind would simply "decide" to swim the English Channel one day. It's understood that such a prodigious undertaking would require an unusually large amount of energy and that no one who hadn't already prepared himself, gaining the strength he needed to do the job, should even attempt it. Let's say a foolish person, not a strong swimmer, did make the attempt. Fatigue would simply overtake him and force him to stop, fatigue being the body's way of quite efficiently and purposefully preventing the creature's death from overexertion.

None of us has ever realized this before, but dieting is the same kind of enterprise. People who are fat are people who haven't been able to extract enough nutrients from their food; the weakness or low fitness level of their tissues is the culprit. When such people go on a diet, they are further weakened by the drop in energy calories the diet provides; more ironically, the body sometimes proceeds to damp down metabolic activity even further in response to diminished nutrient intake. Soon the dieter is experiencing a range of unpleasant reactions (extreme fatigue, grouchiness, excruciating hunger), which is the body's way of saying, "Quit this. This is too strenuous for you, given the metabolic abilities you have at the moment." The person goes off the diet, and gives himself another kick for not having any will power. I need to say it again: the issue is never *moral,* only one of nutritional sufficiency. If you went off your last diet because of one of the symptoms mentioned above, it was because your body wanted you to stop before you got into even greater trouble. Chapter 14 will tell how my doctor, a nutritional specialist, prescribed a regime that improved my digestive abilities simultaneously with losing weight.

Although very few diet books have ever pointed this out, the first phase of any diet should be a repair and buildup phase rather than a "take-it-off" phase. It's no surprise that the books are afraid to mention this; the Type A personality dieters who chronically buy diet books only want to hear how to get that weight off, not how to become healthy. Focused on short-term results, they miss the larger, permanent solution. It's too bad, for they could have the best of both worlds: the unhealthy body almost always contains so much excess water (from the edema of chronic stress or simply excess sodium in the body) that the buildup and unstressing phase always takes off a lot of weight anyway!

This is why the first few days of any diet are usually tolerable, if not downright enjoyable. First, previous binging on carbohydrates has loaded up the liver with glycogen, the stored form of sugar. (Very inefficient metabolizers such as I used to be may take up to four days to use up this supply.) While the glycogen supply lasts, the brain will function normally, for it is still receiving adequate glucose for its needs. Replacing relatively allergenic and stress-inducing binge foods with relatively healthy diet foods will produce a feeling of well-being. A fair amount of weight will be lost, both as cell edema subsides (from the absence of allergens) and as glycogen is finally depleted, which releases sodium, and therefore water.

But as the glycogen is exhausted, the dieter will be less and less capable of handling the diet regime, more and more likely to experience fatigue and mental distress. In his revolutionary book *Nutrition and Your Mind* Dr. George Watson explodes the myth that mental symptoms occurring when the body is under nutritional stress have rational "meaning":

Professor McVay's wife, Isabelle, who wandered out into the night, crying, presents a good example of such psychochemical behavior. Her actions had no meaning ... and resulted solely from impaired energy production in her nervous system. The failure to distinguish between psychochemical behavior and motivated, meaningful behavior is at the bottom of the chaos in psychotherapy. ... Now let us suppose that the abnormal behavior of a person such as Mrs. McVay really consists of meaningless psychochemical responses that are beyond her control, since they are caused by disturbed brain metabolism. Would her behavior change through "talking things over" with a psychotherapist? Hardly. The only way to modify a psychochemical response is to correct the physical processes that are causing it.

The grouchiness and moodiness associated with dieting as we know it is due to the lack of a dependable supply of glucose to the brain. The brain cannot use any fuel *but* glucose (with the exception of ketone bodies in cases of prolonged ketosis, which I will discuss later), and it begins behaving erratically. Watson explains that slow oxidizers (a category which most "lifelong" fat people, at least, fall into) do well on a diet high in carbohydrate-rich proteins (for example, dairy products) or high in protein with some complex carbohydrates added. Since the goal is to keep the supply of glucose to the brain adequate and constant, a slow oxidizer needs to take in carbohydrates (which are metabolized quickly) as interim fuel to keep the brain supplied with glucose before the slowly metabolized proteins become available.

Because they eliminate carbohydrates altogether, the Dr. Stillman and Dr. Atkins types of diet will play havoc with the slow oxidizer's system. I giggle every time I think of Marcia Seligson's wonderful remark: "After two days [on Dr. Stillman's diet] I would kill for an orange." Her body is telling her the truth—craving potassium, glucose, and vitamin C (contained in the orange), it is exerting itself to the utmost to get her to give up this unbalanced regime. (The useful role of Dr. Atkins' diet in permanently reeducating metabolism is discussed a few pages further on.)

So let's say the dieter has found Dr. Atkins' diet too taxing and decides simply to count calories. The lowered calorie total represents a decreased energy supply, so the dieter will feel fatigue. Another double-bind is involved: if the carbohydrate count is not low enough as well, even if calories are low the body will not begin to output FMH, the hypothetical fat-metabolizing hormone. (Anne Scott Beller tells us that this begins to happen only when the carbohydrate count is less than 100 grams per day.) Thus on a simple low-calorie diet a large percentage of the weight lost may actually consist of water and *muscle tissue!* This is why some people reach their ideal weight and still remain too "fat." As David A. Schoenstadt remarks in *The San Francisco Weight Loss Method,* anyone *"can* succeed in losing weight and keeping it off. But not by dieting alone. You can only succeed by increasing your Lean Body Mass, which means improving your physical condition." The muscle-consuming effect is intensified in a total fast; according to George Schauf in *Think Thin,* "Obese seamen who had been starved ten days lost twenty pounds, but it was shown by a radioactive spectrometer and computer that 65 percent, or thirteen pounds, of the weight they had lost while starving was essential vital tissue."

But fat is all we ought to be interested in losing. In *Fat and Thin,* Beller explains that so-called cellulite, the "hard-to-lose" fat, is "the ribbons of connective tissue which serve as pouches for large groups of fat cells. . . . [They lose] their elasticity and shrink with age; the overlying skin which is attached to these fibers then contracts to measure, and . . . a kind of overall dimpling occurs like the dimpling on the surface of a golf ball." The only reason it's "the fat you could never lose before" is that many people go on diets that *don't remove much fat,* just water and muscle.

Given all the double-binds surrounding calorie reduction and food deprivation, a search was inevitable for a diet that would take off fat and still allow adequate calorie intake and adequate nutrition—an approach whose efficacy would derive from persuading the body to set up alternate, more efficient fat-burning metabolic pathways different from the unhealthy ones it was currently using. This would represent a profound and permanent reeducation of the body into a different equilibrium.

There are two schools of thought about weight reduction by means of metabolic changeover or reeducation and how this should best occur; each is (understandably) intolerant of the other. For convenience I will label these two poles of opinion the Atkins Diet (as in *Dr. Atkins' Diet Revolution* or *Dr. Atkins' Superenergy Diet*) and the Pritikin Program (as in *Live Longer Now* and *The Pritikin Program*), though these two men merely represent a larger group of advocates on each side. Dr. Atkins claims that what's wrong with us is hypoglycemia caused by an intolerance for carbohydrates—*all* carbohydrates. On his diet you cut back to zero carbohydrates until you go into ketosis (explained below), then add carbohydrates back into the diet very sparingly (still remaining in ketosis). He says, "This diet *isn't* 'balanced.' It is deliberately *unbalanced.* The reason—to counteract the metabolic imbalance that causes people to get fat in the first place." He claims that he sees people who misguidedly eat high-carbohydrate diets and finds them full of "fatigue or dizziness or tension or drowsiness." You can eat as much as you want of the foods he recommends and still lose weight.

Nathan Pritikin (and others of his opinion, such as Paavo Airola, author of *Hypoglycemia: A Better Approach*) claims that what's wrong with us is hypoglycemia caused by an intolerance for high levels of protein. On his diet you eat 80 percent complex carbohydrates, 10 percent protein, and 10 percent fat. Airola claims that he sees people who misguidedly eat high-protein diets and finds them full of "physical and mental sluggishness, or lack of energy." You can eat large amounts of the foods he recommends and still lose weight.

Whom do we believe? Strange as it sounds, both. Each is recommending a regime that perfectly suits one or the other of the two metabolic poles that Dr. Watson calls "fast and slow oxidizers." Although both these diets are enormously popular because you lose weight on them, both are diets that also attempt to build up the capabilities of the tissues through megavitamin therapy and large amounts of hypoallergenic and nutrient-rich foods, to make the body capable of meeting the energy demands of weight loss.

The Pritikin Program is an eminently sane lifetime eating plan; most people using it will feel a quick and permanent upsurge of health and well-being. Some highly carbohydrate-intolerant people would find after a certain period on the diet that their weight loss was slowing down or ceasing; they would have to start monitoring their carbohydrate intake and perhaps even scale it down until they began to lose again. Though ketosis ought to be temporary rather than permanent, the Atkins Diet can be satisfying too, but it's necessary to explain what goes on with that diet so that the strange symptoms some people experience will no longer seem so mysterious. I am one of those people who practically drop dead on Dr. Atkins' diet. I feel faint or queasy all day, I get heartburn, I snarl at everyone I meet, and so on. In fact, long ago I gave up on it for good; my lifetime eating plan is much closer to the Pritikin Program.

A few years ago my mother was in distress about her weight; she had fifteen extra pounds that she just *couldn't* lose, no matter how hard she tried. She sounded desperate as she told me that, although she continued to eat less and less, nothing seemed to help. There was no suspicion about "sneak eating" secretly boosting her daily calorie total; I knew that if she told me she'd been eating almost nothing, it was the absolute truth. Suddenly something clicked in my brain. She and my father had recently retired and had changed their eating patterns noticeably. I replayed in my mind recent meals I had shared with them and realized that the meals (though very low calorie) were relatively high in natural sugars: granola, dried fruits, and so forth. I trotted out my copy of Dr. Atkins and suggested she use it. After a cursory glance at it she informed me with some severity that she could not possibly bring herself to eat all the food you were supposed to eat on this diet. When I told her that large quantities were not mandatory, but merely a concession to unreformed heavy eaters, she brightened immediately, and took the diet home to try. Three weeks later she joyfully reported that the fifteen pounds simply melted away without a trace, and she had enjoyed every moment of the "diet." Two facts are clear: first, her former diet was too high in carbohydrates for her to lose any weight (whether stored water or fat). Second, as she had never been a slow oxidizer, her brain didn't suffer when carbohydrates were temporarily removed; she thrived on the high-protein regime. She would have made an ideal case for Dr. Atkins' files.

But to get back to people like me—the ones who think they simply can't tolerate this diet. Dr. Atkins is correct when he says that the diet is a great metabolic regulator, but for slow oxidizers the breaking-in period is noticeably taxing, enough to make most people give up. Dr. Atkins' regime represents a forcible attempt to replace one's present equilibrium with a different one. After three weeks or so the body *will* change over, but only after putting up an incredible fight, the intensity of which is, I believe, in direct proportion to the paradoxical carbohydrate dependence/intolerance of one's original metabolism.

In a moment we'll deal with the very real dangers of ketosis, but for now we need to look at it as simply a different metabolic pathway that (from an evolutionary standpoint) once had a survival function. As I said, the time it takes to get fully into ketosis can feel terrible for some people. When carbohydrates are completely absent, ketone bodies substitute for glucose as fuel for the brain; in the three weeks it takes for ketone products to become reliably abundant, it is likely that one will feel intermittently awful: weak, depressed, and so forth. When the ketones do arrive in full force, a kind of euphoria sets in (along with a total absence of hunger) that lasts for the duration of the ketosis.

In one animal experiment rats were force-fed until they were obese and then left to their own devices. The rats voluntarily went on a fast (which produced ketosis) until their weights had once again returned to normal. This indicates that ketosis is not simply some vile scheme perpetrated by an unscrupulous doctor to fleece a gullible public, as some of Dr. Atkins' critics would have us believe. Millions of years ago the food supply was much less sure than it is today; the possibility of prolonged famine was very real. Ketosis is an alternate pathway, a method of mobilizing the body's stored fat and at the same time keeping the creature's mood level and energy level high enough to permit it to make heroic efforts to search for new food supplies. If abilities simply degenerated with lack of food, the process of starvation would run a very predictable course.

Dr. Atkins' diet is billed as a weight-loss diet, though the doctor is least candid with his readers when it comes to explaining the nature of the loss of weight in ketosis. Since ketosis is highly toxic to the body, the kidneys aggressively try to wash away incompletely burned fatty acid molecules and thus minimize the excessively acid state of the body. As they excrete more water than normal, body tissues are dehydrated, and weight is lost—but only temporarily. Fat is lost too, but at a slower rate than the water weight. Edwin Bayrd's book *The Thin Game* is the most stringent exposé to date of the untruths connected with Dr. Atkins' recommendations. It is quite true that if you ate a very high-calorie version of Dr. Atkins' diet for several weeks, then resumed eating carbohydrates the way you used to, nearly all the weight you lost would probably return, because the weight was water forcibly excreted by the kidneys (but which had to be replaced to resume normal health). You would undoubtedly criticize yourself severely for your weight gain, though, again, it would not have been your *fault*—only a reflection of physiological realities.

It goes without saying that the Last Chance Diet (the liquid protein diet) is the most taxing and most toxic kind of ketosis possible. From personal experience I am convinced that the protein-sparing fast used alone is not a wise approach to weight control. (Statistics now show that fifty or so women died as a result of using this method.) I suffered enormous gastric distress at the end of the Lindner Clinic fast, mostly connected with having to reeducate my body in how to digest food. The last time I inquired, the clinic was using what they called a daylight fast—two meals of liquid protein plus a well-balanced dinner (which provides, among other things, natural potassium and some roughage).

Water retention is a perennial worry to dieters, though the diuretics used as a "solution" are worse than the original problem. The widespread use of diuretics is inevitable in a Type A society whose overweight members lust for results, though a more classic example of the you-push-one-way, your-body-pushes-back tendency could scarcely be imagined. Your body is now retaining water, usually because you are eating a diet that is too high in sodium. According to Dr. Alberto Cormillot in *Thin Forever,* when you take a diuretic to get rid of your puffiness, "this elimination [of water] causes a metabolic change in the composition of the blood, and the adrenal glands (which always try to maintain an equilibrium) immediately produce a substance called aldosterone, which attempts to halt the loss of sodium by retaining it, together with water." The body would not contain excess water in the first place if you ate a more largely vegetarian diet richer in potassium. Furthermore, such a diet would cause your body to maintain proper "tissue turgor" (the major cause of sagging skin following weight loss is the lack of turgor produced by too-rapid excretion of water). Stupidly, some people even decrease their liquid intake while dieting to make the scale reading more acceptable. Focusing on short-term results—a pound or two lost—blinds them to the long-term drawbacks of droopy flesh.

The water-retention issue brings up another possible area of major imbalance in the unhealthy body: that between sodium and potassium. It works this way: the stress response by the adrenal glands includes the output of cortisol and aldosterone, both antidiuretic hormones, that is, ones causing the retention of sodium (and water) and the excretion of potassium. A given concentration of potassium in the cells is balanced by a given concentration of sodium outside the cells. Since the balance between sodium and potassium is governed by the body's homeostatic mechanisms, an untoward increase in sodium causes the retention of water to dilute it to the proper level. An increase in sodium, furthermore, softens cell walls and permits potassium to leave the cells and be excreted. But cellular potassium is vital to the proper utilization of glucose; without it the body cannot maintain proper blood sugar levels (and lowered blood sugar levels initiate stress, further exacerbating the sodium-retention potassium-deficiency problem). As I said earlier, a largely vegetarian (potassium-rich) diet will improve the functioning of any hypoglycemic. We do not need to eat anything like the amount of salt we have become habituated to. The fine structure of our archaic bodies was designed for a diet plentiful in potassium and very scarce in sodium; there are abundant mechanisms to conserve the body's sodium (reabsorption by the kidney tubules, for example) and just as many to waste its potassium.

It is worthwhile to mention here another cause for the wide variety of results people experience on Dr. Atkins' diet. The foods you are allowed to eat in unlimited quantities are: fats; protein foods such as meat, eggs, and cheese; and vegetables. The high-calorie permitted foods (butter, cheese, salted nuts, etc.) are very high in sodium, and their excessive use would aggravate the overacidity of ketosis (whose other name is *acidosis*) and thus put the body under even greater stress. A person who chose meals from the low-calorie, vegetable (that is, generally potassium-rich) side of the permitted list would probably have much less difficulty.

As Chapter 6 mentioned, mimicking is the way a processed or artificial substance elicits the same response as one of the body's natural substances, which leads to a mistaken craving for the former. Stimulants such as nicotine and caffeine mimic adrenalin's effects in the body. I was told at the Lindner Clinic that chocolate mimics the effect of estrogen in the body, which is why many women (including myself) crave chocolate premenstrually: the body has just undergone a rapid drop in estrogen level and is trying, mistakenly, to restore its previous balance. (Again, cravings such as these are not a *moral* issue, but a biochemical one.)

Hearing messages from our body with any accuracy requires being more attentive than most of us are accustomed to. We need to trust our instincts more than before, though we also need to realize that lower animals have it easy by comparison, since their instincts are hard-wired in the brain, making it impossible for them to make mistakes. (As Lewis Thomas jokes, "Fish are flawless in everything they do.") Our power of choice unfortunately implies the ability to make bad choices—a privilege we have recently been exercising to a life-threatening degree. I highly approve of Dr. John Yudkin's remark, "If you eat the right *sorts* of food, you will automatically eat the right *amounts* of food," because it stresses the automatic nature of good behavior. My aim has always been to try to find the method "closest to play"—that is, the most effortless path, which is effortless because it cooperates with the way things automatically work.

As you increase your intuitiveness and sophistication in interpreting feedback, you will inevitably learn to appreciate the virtues of styles of life other than our own—what might be called cultural alternate pathways. As members of an "advanced" technological society, we are highly prone to dismiss any less "advanced" society's solutions to common problems (particularly nutrition) as naive or unscientific. The evidence is mounting, however, that it is *we*, not they, who are on the wrong track. Nathan Pritikin commented in a *New York Times Book Review* interview, "There are only two diets in the world—the Western diet, which has half of its total calories in fat and is also high in cholesterol, and the diet of underdeveloped countries, which has one-fifth the fat and one-tenth the cholesterol."

For example, the Oriental notion of balancing meals using the principles of yin and yang may seem to the uninitiated an esoteric discipline embodying highly arbitrary categories. Not so; when you eat according to yin and yang complementarity, you present to the body a balanced mixture of food in harmony with the pH and concentration of the body's own fluids (which food therefore minimizes stress). In questions of nutrition yin and yang, which have no precise "scientific" definition, correspond to alkalinity (primarily potassium) and acidity (primarily sodium), together with the diluting effect of water. Yin represents the principle of expansion—things growing, getting bigger, absorbing water. Fruits are especially yin, and melons among the most yin of all. Yang represents the principle of contraction—shrinking, removing the water, compressing. Cheese, for example, is a compressed (more yang) version of milk; meat is more yang than all the grass that went into making it. Refined sugar and salt in large amounts are so excessively yin and yang, respectively, that they are considered harmful to the body. A truly knowledgeable disciple of macrobiotics would undoubtedly find this truncated summary of the complexities of yin and yang amusing and even a bit ludicrous; it is not necessary, however, for you to become a strict devotee of macrobiotics in order to use these principles intelligently in your eating. Someone taking yin and yang into account as he ate would, without knowing it, be acting according to highly respected physiochemical principles.

George Ohsawa once observed, "Macrobiotic eating gives us a bodily condition which helps us express gratitude," a statement that fits intimately with Dr. Selye's remark that an attitude of thanksgiving is the primary antistress emotion. Ohsawa is correct at the biochemical level; stress-free eating removes the barriers to a grateful state of mind. In fact, when the body is right, gratitude does not have to be *willed*; it comes of its own accord. *Cooking for Life* and *Cooking with Care and Purpose* by Michel Abehsera provide a useful, highly readable introduction to the subject. *Diet for a Small Planet* by Frances Moore Lappé and *Recipes for a Small Planet* by Ellen Buchman Ewald are other useful books of a similar kind.

The whole name of the game is better, more sensitive balance for the body. When your tissues are healthy and you are eating right, your brain is well-nourished and you feel fine. You hear it so often it's become a truism, but it's true nonetheless: good health is the most valuable possession any of us will ever have. Our body tries its best to keep us in good health; when we willingly cooperate, our chances for attaining and maintaining that state are increased many times over.

14
A New, Healthy Body –
From the Inside Out

Knowledge cannot be separated from a certain way of
life which becomes its living manifestation.
          Fritjof Capra, *The Tao of Physics*

This chapter, more than any other, could be called the "nuts and
bolts," the instructions for what to do. But these instructions are the
least important part of what I have to say; I've included them more as
reminders than anything else, so you won't miss some important part
of the complex total as you start out on your own journey toward lifelong thinness and health. I have also included many references to
books that treat each of these separate topics in more detail than I
could; consult them if you find yourself stymied by the lack of one specific bit of knowledge. I believe that this book's greatest value will be
to help you *see the whole;* after you've done that, the rest of the
instructions (*anyone's* instructions) will be relatively simple to carry
out.

The instructions in this chapter are arranged in a way that corre-
sponds roughly to the priority order I mentioned in Chapter 1. With
the hope that this book has already helped to ameliorate the unworkable view of reality that is the largest part of the problem, the other
groupings shade from "Relieving Anxiety" into "Improving Chemistry" and "Changing Habits."

A few words about obstacles and resistances are in order. Both are
very real, and until you at least acknowledge the ones you have, you
can't hope to get anywhere. At various times in my life I have felt as if
obstacle was my middle name; if I listed all the obstacles I've encoun-
tered in my lifelong search for thinness, this book would easily be fifty
pages longer than it is. Obstacles are like knots: they are composed of
many strands, and the only way to get through them is to pick at them

patiently, a strand at a time, not to take to them with a butcher knife. Anger or impatience are inappropriate—they just don't do the trick.

As earlier chapters have stated, wherever you are at this moment is *your* starting point. The "facts" about your condition don't matter in the least; it makes no difference if you have two hundred pounds to lose, or five. You simply *are:* right there at square one. There's absolutely nothing wrong with where you are now, either. My own decision to eat properly is, contrary to all our culture's beliefs, not something I *do;* it's something I *am.* A "doing" would be a performance; this is an expression of my being. Whenever you bring yourself to eat sensibly, you are in some sense practicing further good behavior, but if your sensible eating is a "diet" (and we all agree that the most important part of a "diet" is going off it), then your "I-am-so-deprived" state of mind will cancel most of the benefits of the good behavior. As Don Juan says in Castaneda's *A Separate Reality,* "The indulgence of denying is by far the worst; it forces us to believe we are doing great things."

The first big obstacle to face is wanting the goal but resisting the idea of the lifelong good behavior required to get there. I can profoundly empathize with this feeling. (I *ought* to be able to; I experienced it continuously for twenty-five years.) My only counsel is to remember that all your conscious thoughts are only artifacts of the state of your body's health; first allow your body to become fully healthy, then check back to see what your thoughts are. Willingness has a nutritional component. I found that my definitions of what food was alluring and what was distasteful changed remarkably after my body became healthy; as Proust wrote, "We do not succeed in changing things according to our desire, but gradually our desire changes." It is also extremely important to understand that what I call lifelong good behavior does not mean spending the rest of your life in a straitjacket—that is too unpleasant even to contemplate. The world is here to enjoy. But there is an enormous difference between the way a healthy body and an unhealthy one react to food. I find that I can occasionally eat something the fat me would have thought extremely wicked, and do so without noticeable effect. Most of my food used to be junk food, with occasional forays into healthy eating; now it's by far the other way around.

The second obstacle to perfect serenity during weight loss, which I also profoundly empathize with, is impatience over the passage of time. It's such a natural attitude for us in the Western world that I'm at a loss to tell you how to avoid it; all I can say is that I found my own crazy impatience fading away the healthier and thinner I became. Reich says in *From Fat to Skinny,* "Often when someone tells me, 'I want to lose fifty pounds. How long will it take?' my only answer can be, 'As long as it does.'" He adds, "You cease to dwell on time, and therefore time does not become a barrier."

So now here are the instructions. The first two are absolutely crucial; they are those that most other diet books gloss over or ignore. They and the third represent the three most important kinds of *fitness training*—for that is the best description of it—in the areas where we are now underexercised and flabby and need remedial help to get back to normal function so that we can adequately cope with the stresses our life provides. The first of these is relaxation/meditation, the second digestion, and the third cardiovascular exercise.

RELAXATION/MEDITATION

As Chapter 6 observed, *relaxation* ordinarily refers to getting rid of tensions in the body, *meditation* to relieving those in the mind. Because we are bodyminds, we need both. Meditation practice is mentioned first both because of its direct connection with feelings of serenity and because your relaxation/meditation program ought to be running fairly smoothly in your life *before* you take on the other major job of losing weight. Trying to adjust to both at the same time might be unnecessarily difficult. A meditative state of mind is essential for many of the specific "doings" mentioned earlier in the book: mantras, visualizations, even physical exercise. Meditative consciousness is not limited to closing your eyes and keeping quiet for fifteen minutes morning and evening. Your daily practice merely shows you what a serene state of mind feels like; you then try to maintain that state all during the day. José Silva defines the right mental state to use all day long as "that feeling you get when things are working," a feeling of positive expectancy. As mentioned earlier, the best basic book is Benson's *The Relaxation Response.* Another entertaining variation, which can sometimes also bring about unexpected insights, is the "mind trips" concept invented by Frances Stern and Ruth Hoch in *Mind Trips to Help You Lose Weight.*

DIGESTIVE FITNESS

When Dr. An Thanh asked me, on my first visit to his office, whether I evacuated every day, I felt like replying indignantly, "Certainly not!" To me a daily bowel movement was something I was ashamed of when it happened, since it always meant that I had eaten so much food the previous day that my body had to work overtime to process it all. It had never been explained to me that daily elimination was the most important index of digestive fitness; not only the volume of food, but also the competence of one's intestinal flora, determine how often one eliminates. Less than once a day indicates subnormal digestive fitness. Dr. An Thanh examined my tongue (coated), which confirmed his diagnosis. Thankfully, the condition is very simple to correct: Dr. An Thanh asked me to take two lactobacillus-acidophilus-plus-pectin capsules and a chewable papaya enzyme tablet after each meal; after dinner I also chewed a tablespoon of cooked azuki bean, a small red Japanese bean (optional). I was thankful he didn't ask me to take brewer's yeast; however, it would have helped in the same way. I also began on his recommended food plan, which included lots of cooked and raw vegetables and a cup or more of brown rice daily. Very quickly my digestion improved enormously, and therefore my ability to absorb nutrients from food did too. As a result, my moods went from erratic to predominantly sunny and happy, and my body even got warmer, since my better nourished tissues were producing more heat. This alteration in itself was enough to change my equilibrium from a deranged, unstable one with great weight fluctuations into a highly stable one in which I don't gain weight as a result of what I eat.

Please understand that "good digestion" has nothing to do with how well one "tolerates" food (I always said I had a cast iron stomach). It is also not a condition that can be improved by means of antacids. Hyperacidity contributes to the problem, of course, for an over-acid environment is unhealthy for the body as a whole. But antacid preparations only attempt to mask an uncomfortable symptom, rather than treat the real cause—the excess acidity of the average Western diet.

As I observed in Chapter 13, one of our cultural blind spots is that in our minds we separate health-building food regimes from weight-loss diets. Nothing could be more foolish; fat people actually need health building *more* than other people. But everyone needs good digestion; in *Your Body Is Your Best Doctor* Dr. Melvin Page estimates that most of the population operates at between 40 percent and 70 percent of the desirable level of digestive efficiency. Digestive fitness is the key to the breakthrough I promised in Chapter 1: the true First Step that everyone else leaves out, and the only lasting cornerstone of genuinely permanent, stress-free weight loss.

CARDIOVASCULAR EXERCISE

From personal experience I'm quite sure that this task will be hardest of all to make happen effortlessly in your life. Though three weeks is always mentioned as the standard time to habituate various sorts of mental and physical behavior, George Leonard says of running in *The Ultimate Athlete,* "The first weeks are the hardest. You will definitely start noticing a difference after six weeks of training." Overweight people also have to cope with natural negative feelings about being seen in public huffing and puffing (which is not required; simply begin with a walking program). But remember Dr. Schoenstadt, author of *The San Francisco Weight-Loss Method,* remarked that he failed four times before he made his exercise program a continuing part of his life; and that the only way to be successful on a diet is not to cut calories alone, but also to increase the body's muscle mass through exercise. Remember also Dr. Lamb's point that exercise seems to activate fat-burning rather than fat-storing metabolic pathways. (It also seems to stimulate metabolic action by anywhere from 10 to 28 percent for as much as fifteen hours after the end of the exercise.) Covert Bailey's *Fit or Fat?* is an absolutely first-rate and highly detailed account of how to determine the right amount of exercise for you and the rate at which you should progress.

But the recommendation of exercise goes far beyond the agreeable benefits for one's figure. Perhaps the most significant benefit of sustained cardiovascular exercise is that it induces a calm, meditative state of mind as well. Dr. Arnold Mandell, a neurologist with a compelling personal interest in exercise physiology, observed in an interview that running increases right-brain dominance, which is associated with increased levels of alpha waves. After ten minutes or so of jogging, levels of serotonin (a "serenity" substance in the brain) rise noticeably. In *The Thin Book* Jeanne Eddy Westin reports the results of a study in which anxious subjects were divided into three groups: one group jogged, one did nothing, and the third both jogged and meditated. As might be expected, the third group experienced the greatest reduction in anxiety levels. When I run, I often repeat to myself a continuous mantra, which both focuses my attention and distracts me from my initial resistance to exercising. I change the mantra from day to day, depending on what I feel like expressing.

For those who know they will never succeed in their "search for their inner athlete," as George Leonard puts it, because they could never learn to like being out of breath, perhaps the best words are those of Fred Rohé: "Don't overdo it. Underdo it. You aren't running because you're in a hurry to get somewhere. You will be able to run tirelessly if you follow this simple rule: Run *within* your breath, do not run *ahead* of your breath." He also counsels moderation: "Thinking you can run around the block, just run down to the corner." The key, Rohé says, "is always to do less than you think you can."

MEDICAL TESTS; IDENTIFYING ALLERGIES

If your doctor prescribes a glucose tolerance test for you, make sure that it is at least a five-hour, not a three-hour, test. For several years my gynecologist listened to my complaints and sent me off annually for another three-hour glucose tolerance test, only to announce brightly, "Your test results are normal, Mrs. Bryan; there's nothing wrong with you." At the Lindner Clinic I had my first five-hour test, which showed a precipitous drop in blood sugar level at the fourth hour; I was a classic hypoglycemic, but the shorter tests hadn't been able to detect it. As Chapter 6 mentioned, sometimes the early part of the test curve seems normal merely because the hypoglycemic may also be a slow oxidizer; in other words, his metabolism works on the glucose slowly and inefficiently, keeping his blood sugar high at first. Only later does the insulin overreaction make his blood sugar level plummet.

Finding out if you have any food allergies, which is necessary to ensure stress-free eating, is mostly a matter of trial and error. The most expensive way to do it is via the classic allergy tests in a doctor's office. You may discover previously unsuspected allergies as you search for the best way of eating for you. When you cut out salt and sugar, the biggest stressors, the messages from the allergens unique to you will, in the absence of the other stress factors, become louder and clearer. Dr. An Thanh's food recommendations for me excluded milk and wheat products, and for the first time in my life I discovered that I had been allergic to these all along. I then realized that one of my constant problems in dieting was that although I ate smaller quantities of food, I was still eating the foods I was allergic to and was therefore still experiencing the stress response in its undiminished form. Four books that can be of great help in pinpointing individual food allergy/reactivity are *Dr. Newbold's Revolutionary New Discoveries about Weight Loss, Dr. Mandell's Five-Day Allergy Relief System,* Arthur Coca's *The Pulse Test,* and Dr. Arthur Kaslow's wonderful book, *Freedom From Chronic Disease.*

CALCULATING IDEAL WEIGHT

Although all of us love height-weight tables (they're something of a national pastime), they are not accurate enough for our purposes; generalized charts such as these don't cover an adequately diverse range of body type and composition. As the June 4, 1979, issue of *Sporting Times* stated, "It is possible for two people to be 40 pounds apart in weight and have totally different body types, yet be the same in terms of body fat." To realistically determine how much weight you need to lose, you need to find out your ideal weight (a number unique to you). This means determining your fat-free weight, then adding a percentage of that figure (20 percent for women, 15 percent for men) to arrive at your ideal weight.

To do this you will need either access to a YMCA that will do the measurements for you or one of the following books or magazine articles. *Getting in Shape* by Frank Katch, William McArdle and Brian R. Boylan goes into great detail about how to measure your own percentage of body fat. The January 1978 issue of *Mademoiselle* contains a calculation system for determining women's fat percentages. At the back of Charles Kuntzleman's *Activetics* there are cardboard calipers you can use to take skinfold measurements and a chart to help you interpret them.

Figuring out how long your weight loss ought to take has diabolical temptations toward Type A rushing of the process; be as conservative as you possibly can. In *Think Slim—Be Slim* Elyse Birkinshaw suggests setting three goals: the first week, halfway through, and final goal. In *Thin Forever* Dr. Alberto Cormillot gives an interesting rule of thumb: "You can hope to lose approximately two to three percent of your weight in the first week, one to one and one-half percent of your weight during each additional week." Your weight loss will *seem* more acceptable to you at first, when it's accompanied by the loss of water, though later, smaller losses represent just as large a loss of fat as before.

The various types of overweight people will experience various degrees of difficulty in losing weight. The luckiest, of course, are those who are primarily retaining excess water (like my mother, in Chapter 13); all they have to do is eat fewer carbohydrates for a while and they will automatically reach their goal weight. Losing is next easiest for those whose body chemistry is basically sound but who have simply allowed themselves a few too many bad habits for too long a time (like my husband, in Chapter 3). The worst off are the true compulsive eaters (like me), who have a deranged metabolism and a physiological addiction as well as all the problems of the other two types. They can be helped with a healing, stress-free diet and a meditative discipline. But remember: *everyone can succeed.*

SUPPORT

Everyone does better with loving support, whether from an individual (see *The Love Diet Strategy*) or an organization (TOPS, Weight Watchers, or Overeaters Anonymous). The advantage of the love diet strategy is that the trusted friend (the "feeder") takes care of the burden of planning the dieter's meals, which automatically removes much of the anxiety connected with choosing one's food. Reporting your planned food intake to a trusted friend every day for a least a month (the basis of the beginner's program in Overeaters Anonymous) would be of enormous help in getting through the period in which you were becoming habituated to new behavior and in which your equilibrium was changing to a healthier one.

Weight Watchers is a multimillion-dollar-a-year business. Its diet, based on the New York City Public Health Department's weight-loss plan, is sound, though needlessly and arbitrarily regimented. In a sense, it encourages a certain unhealthy obsession with food (distinct from relaxed, serenity-promoting mindfulness). But perhaps the greatest visible drawback to Weight Watchers (which may be offset by the rewards of group experience and sharing) is its emphasis on performance and its chastisement of people who gain instead of lose. A very affecting tale of the excruciating performance anxiety associated with being a Weight Watchers instructor is told by Leslie Maynard in her book *The Freedom Diet*.

FINDING THE BEST DIET

This part of the process could be immediate, because you simply pick up one of your old favorite diets and are successful with it, or take a long time, because your new knowledge makes all your old diets' shortcomings too obvious. The right one will have to be *your* discovery; all I can do is make some recommendations about what worked well for me. Working with a nutritionist to devise a personalized plan for you would make the trial-and-error process less random and therefore less time-consuming. Consumer Guide's *Rating the Diets* presents a great deal of useful information. My present eating program, which I plan to continue for the rest of my life, is basically very similar to the Pritikin Program: low in fat, medium in protein, and high in vegetables and complex carbohydrates (grains and fruits). I am not a fanatic anything: vegetarian, diet faddist, vitamin freak, whatever. As I said earlier in this chapter, my new healthy digestive system lets me "get away with" very occasional indulgences into tempting foods with almost no punishment other than not feeling quite as well as usual.

Yvonne Young Tarr's wonderful book *The Ten-Minute Gourmet Diet Cookbook*, despite its comic title, is one of the best accounts available of the way someone with a weight problem can find the right diet empirically, discovering by trial and error what does and does not work for her body. I like her eating plan, too, because it uses to good advantage the body's own cyclical nature. Her "Fat-Scat Plan" is basically one week of counting calories alternating with one week of counting carbohydrates. Dr. Barbara Edelstein's *The Woman Doctor's*

Diet for Women is also excellent, and highly detailed in its explanations of specifically female weight-loss problems.

FOOD CALCULATIONS

Losing weight is a complex problem in thermodynamics. An engineer would never try to solve this kind of problem without understanding the theoretical principles that governed it, and you shouldn't have to, either. But even with all the millions of different "diets" and "fat-burning foods" that are claimed to exist, the underlying weight-loss equations, or principles, are simple enough to understand. The only thing a dieter wants to lose is *fat tissue*. It is not desirable to lose either water (except the water from edema, which will come off by itself) or lean tissue (since this will simply replace itself when the diet is over). From the latter point of view, a low-calorie diet makes more sense than fasting. As Beller remarks in *Fat and Thin*, "in some patients on an 800-calorie-a-day diet, real fat loss was actually greater than it was on a regime of total fasting. . . . with a bare minimum of nutrients coming into the system from time to time, the brain can still make do . . . and the body's protein stores need not get called into action for emergency glucose deliveries to the brain. Fat will thus be burned for fuel, and lean tissue spared."

To make sure that the largest possible percentage of your weight loss actually *is* fat, your diet must be simultaneously low in calories, low in carbohydrates, adequate in protein, and high in vitamins, minerals, water, and roughage. Yes—it's got to be all of them. And that's the double-bind: the "high-protein" allowance recommended on many diets may also be so high in calories that loss of fat proceeds only very slowly. The protein-sparing fast would be an ideal solution to the enough-protein/low-calorie requirement if it weren't for its devastating practical drawbacks. The Lindner Clinic assigned me 75 grams of liquid protein daily—a total of 300 calories—assuming that this much would "spare" my lean tissue and allow cell repair. (This now seems too much protein to me.) Liquid protein has 1 protein gram for each 4 calories, or a ratio of 1 to 4. Using a simple calorie and food composition chart, you could carry out a similar calculation for all the protein foods your food plan includes, then favor those that approach liquid protein's 1-to-4 ratio. (Shrimp, many kinds of fish, and poultry are nearly the same, and some soy protein powder supplements might come close.)

The only joyful news I can report is that, on the basis of my own experience, most people will be delighted to realize just how much of their excess weight is excess water held in the tissues because of improper food choices (allergenic foods and too much sugar and salt). At the beginning of my diet I could eat relatively large portions of brown rice and still lose relatively large amounts of weight. The weight loss slowed as I got halfway to my goal, and the rest proceeded more or less according to conventional diet wisdom (low calorie, low carbohydrate). By then, however, I had become habituated to the healthy food, and eating smaller quantities was relatively easy.

VITAMINS, MINERALS, AND WATER

Forget what the doctors tell us about how Americans have the most vitamin-rich urine in the world. As I argued in Chapter 13, many obese people are undernourished, and a program of remedial vitamins is crucial to recovery. The entire complex of B vitamins, for example, is important to someone who has been a sugar addict, since sugar is an antinutrient, consuming the body's store of B vitamins in the process of its own digestion. Anyone who has been under chronic stress from a poor diet needs to take large, continuous daily amounts of vitamin C (the antistress vitamin) as well. Hypoglycemics who have difficulty avoiding the hungry-tired syndrome should consider taking 500 mg. of vitamin C together with two fructose tablets whenever fatigue threatens, so as to keep the blood sugar level high enough to avoid the onset of the stress response. Niacinamide is another vitamin that has shown results in alleviating the symptoms of hypoglycemia. Iodine helps stimulate the thyroid gland and therefore the rate of cell activity; some enzymes also use it for their functioning. A calcium supplement may also be advisable (getting adequate calcium may be more difficult if you are allergic to milk). Books that can help you evaluate the proper amounts and proportions of vitamins for your needs are Adelle Davis' *Let's Eat Right to Keep Fit*, George Watson's *Nutrition and Your Mind*, Cheraskin and Ringsdorf's *Psychodietetics*, and Richard Passwater's *Supernutrition*. *Dr. Atkins' Superenergy Diet* also contains materials on megavitamin therapy.

Water intake is particularly important when losing weight. Beller tells us, "The advice to drink plenty of water while you are on a diet is therefore well taken . . . because whatever works to preserve fat stores in the body seems closely calibrated to whatever it is that also conserves water." By now we've all heard that it's necessary to drink at least eleven glasses of water a day on the ketotic diets (which is why they are sometimes dubbed the "water diet"). This amount of water washes out vitamins at a great rate, though; be careful to replace them. Even if you are not on a ketosis-based diet, when you burn fat you will inevitably dip into ketosis now and then, perhaps many times in a day. Because of this, your blood will tend to be more acid than normal, so drink enough water to keep the acidity diluted and eat potassium-rich foods to return your system to the right balance. Regularizing your blood pH, your potassium intake, and the water balance of your tissues would all occur automatically if you increased your daily consumption of vegetables. These foods are high in water, rich in natural nutrients, and—when eaten raw—good sources of enzymes.

DISCIPLINE AND MINDFULNESS

Chapters 7 and 8 argued the virtues of discipline as the orderly progress toward a goal. Sticking to a disciplined plan, no matter what it is, can be a stress-reducing experience; as a friend once remarked to me, "I think of discipline as doing something worthy of praise." Naturally, we all feel better about ourselves when we've just done something praiseworthy.

Mindfulness is merely being deliberate and careful enough to sustain the discipline. Whenever I think of mindfulness I think of my three-year-old daughter carrying a mug full of milk to the table—deliberation and concentration personified. Mindfulness and attention are Zen notions, though of course they are not limited to Zen. One of the best-known behavior modification principles is to make eating your sole activity; when you do that, you're automatically pursuing your "doing" with mindfulness and attention.

You've heard many times, "When you're on a diet, don't try to do a lot of other things at the same time." That's true. But, paradoxically, one of the principles of Gallwey's Inner Game is that you foster serenity when you become fascinatedly and mindfully absorbed in something else besides the tennis game, the diet, whatever. Many of Gallwey's Inner Game exercises have you do something, anything, to get the mind focused outside itself. You can't feel anxiety if you're absorbed and focused. Whatever you choose—an old hobby, a new hobby, a vocation—it should be something that you can work away at without performance anxiety, since that would be self-defeating Glasser explains in *Positive Addiction* that pastimes producing positive addiction are always something to pursue alone, without competition. With the right degree of concentration on something else, dieting can be made to disappear from your conscious mind, which lets your bodymind carry on with its work unimpeded.

BODY AWARENESS

Body awareness progresses simultaneously with improvements in self-image. Body awareness has been stifled in overweight people; their bodies are the major area in which they "disown" themselves. I had a severe problem along these lines; I was never particularly well-coordinated, so I never learned to appreciate my body for either its performance or its appearance. Friends with weight problems similar to mine never seemed to suffer quite as much as I did, either because they once had respected their bodies or because they weren't as neurotic as I was about my problems.

One of the first steps toward overcoming the estrangement between me and my body was the Progoff Intensive Journal Workshop. Among the exercises we did was a Dialogue with the Body, in which we were to write down the major milestones in our body's life (a sort of preliminary rehearsal of its history), then write a dialogue with our body concerning some current problem—with us writing both sides. The things I wrote down when my "body" was speaking absolutely astonished me, and I learned a good deal. Progoff's book *At a Journal Workshop* contains a moving passage about an aging woman's dialogue with her body:

"It used to be," she told her body, "that any old rag I had would look beautiful on you. But now I can hardly find a dress big enough to fit you." ... "If you still want to be beautiful," her body told her, "you can't count on me. You'll have to find some other way to be beautiful." And with that wisdom to guide her, laughing and serious, she could say YES to the transitions of her age.

There are several books that could be used at home to foster body awareness, among them Moshe Feldenkrais' *Awareness Through Movement*, Wilfred Barlow's *The Alexander Technique*, Thérèse Bertherat's *The Body Has Its Reasons*, Sarah Barker's *The Alexander Technique*: *The Revolutionary Way to Use Your Body for Total Energy*, and Robert Masters and Jean Houston's *Listening to the Body*.

RECORDING FEELINGS

This stress-reducing tool is extremely important. For ongoing serenity you need to learn how to feel your emotions, accept them, and discharge them from your mind and muscles. Behavior therapy always starts with writing down what you eat, though quite clearly the food you eat is secondary to the feelings you've had that have made you *want* to eat. First learn to record your feeling states, then record your food. I kept a food journal a while ago, but I left a space after every entry where I could write down "frustration," "boredom," or "anxiety" if I was feeling any of them. Many of my binges were connected in some way to one of those three emotions; *they* were what needed changing before I could proceed.

You may be curious as to how anyone can stay serene under the stress of the daily vicissitudes of family life. The best method available is still to write down the emotions you feel and thereby neutralize them. Raysa Rose Bonow provides fairly detailed directions in *How to Be a Thin Person* for dealing firmly with family members whose own eating preferences are sabotaging yours. Laurence Reich's *From Fat to Skinny* contains a priceless imaginary dialogue with his Aunt Elly, who is trying to derail his diet with fiendishly delicious homemade pastries.

There are only two kinds of eating: to satisfy hunger, and to provide for other needs. Theodore Isaac Rubin says in *Forever Thin*, "We meet obese people who see and feel food as love, warmth, comfort, security, reward, stimulation, sedation, sex, and many other things." When I overate, I did so because equally satisfying ways to fill my other needs were not readily available. Remember also the man I mentioned in Chapter 11 who told me he had finally learned to seek out the affection he needed rather than drown that need in food.

RECORDING EATING BEHAVIOR

You can tell I'm no behaviorist; recording behavior is fairly low on my list of priorities. But while I'm convinced that the truly significant issues lie in biochemical areas, I also agree that attention to behavior—if done in the proper spirit of serenity—is a good tool for increasing awareness of *what is*.

The things we've learned and become proficient at we perform by means of incredibly complex and sophisticated feedback mechanisms, all operating subliminally. We have forgotten how we do the things we know how to do; we just do them. Because, being ashamed of them, we don't like to look at our out-of-control eating episodes, we never allow ourselves to learn anything about how we really act. I was astounded after a few weeks of recording my behavior faithfully to discover that what I *really* did had no relation whatever to what I *thought* I did. I once thought my binging was spread out equally all through the day and night. Not so: it was overwhelmingly concentrated in the afternoon, from about 2 P.M. until dinnertime. The morning was only a minor problem by comparison, and I almost never overate after dinner, probably more out of a fear of family censure than anything else. Once I found out when I really did eat, I could be more effective at devising strategies to make sure I wouldn't eat. Writing it all down is a way of starting to identify chains of behavior, too—those predispositions to eat that start far before the binge comes on (Richard Stuart mentions these in *Act Thin, Stay Thin*, as does Dorothy Tennov in *Super Self*).

Research has shown that there are marked differences between obese mind-set eaters and normal eaters. Overeaters are people who do things like the following: eat more if food is readily available; eat until the food is gone (that is, don't stop when full); eat faster; take larger bites; eat without pausing. Now that I know (and can admit) I'm this type of eater and am therefore prone to eat when I see food rather than waiting until I'm truly hungry, I simply keep tempting things out of the house or out of my sight in a tall cupboard. I have

even been known to ask my husband to hide certain impossibly alluring things out in the garage.

Always, each separate part of a person's behavior fits with, and can
be explained by reference to, the whole of his or her personality. I used
to fret about the instructions in the behavior modification books to eat
slowly; I found that instruction harder to follow than any of the others, such as eat in one place only, or never eat while standing up. I finally saw that fast eating was simply an isolated instance of my general too-fast approach to life. (I have never been successful at changing
my rate of eating; I will probably always shovel in food at a too-rapid
rate. But since I no longer eat too much food as a result of eating too
rapidly, I no longer worry about it very much. Some day I may learn
how to eat slowly, though I wouldn't bet on it.)

REFINING EATING BEHAVIOR

When your out-of-control behavior has subsided somewhat, you
may want to continue learning about yourself and your behavior. Two
books are invaluable for this exploration: the Pearsons' *The Psychologist's Eat-Anything Diet Book* and Gerrard's *One Bowl*. Both describe
an ongoing process of discovery about eating in harmony with one's
natural preferences. I did not describe them earlier in the section on
how to select a diet because anyone who is still functioning primarily
as an addict will not be able to use "food awareness" approaches, for
his or her body is not yet generating meaningful feedback about food
preferences. First you need to repair your digestive equipment; then
you can talk meaningfully of likes and dislikes.

Gerrard makes it clear that refining his eating behavior meant becoming more exquisitely aware of all the signals his body was sending
him. Some of these could be heard only if he slowed down the eating
process and became more attentive to small signals from his body.
One well-known behavior modification suggestion is to pause and wait
in the middle of a meal. This has a very sound basis in the physiology
of digestion. It takes up to twenty minutes for the body to signal that
it's full; a fast eater consuming easy-to-eat high-calorie food could
have eaten much more than his body wanted by that time, before his
body could manage to say, "Enough."

THE JOURNEY, NOT THE ARRIVAL, MATTERS

Ideally, a diet should be a time of such gradual personal evolution that the goal arrives without being distinguishable from the effort itself. As Dr. Henry A. Jordan says in *Eating is Okay!*, "The day you reach your ultimate weight goal should be no different for you than the day before." This will be particularly true if you've been allowing yourself to have experiences that make you feel as good as if you were thin even before you get there.

An advertisement for Kretschmer wheat germ proclaims, "If you take care of the inside, the inside will take care of the outside." This is a very good life motto for those of us trying to stay serene in order to stay slim. Jeanne Eddy Westin says in *The Thin Book* something we all need to hear as we try for daily serenity: "Each day is related to our life as a brick is related to a house. Each day is a whole day and stands alone, and yet each one supports the other days that go to make up the years of our lives."

Laurence LeShan once wrote a moving note complimenting his wife Eda LeShan (the author of *Winning the Losing Battle*) after she had lost a great deal of weight but was still feeling dissatisfied. Part of it went as follows: "The finest thing a human being can do—and the hardest—is to grow past our own special enemy, the traitor within, and become free of it." This is our goal, and it *can* be reached. I hope this book helps you see the way.

Afterword:
Social Reverberations

For the point where I am most myself I am most beyond
myself. At root I am one with all the other branches.
Alan Watts, quoted in *The Gospel According to Zen*

Losing weight is the only self-improvement endeavor in which achieving the goal requires not only the decision to stop the undesirable behavior but also the passage of a good deal of time. A smoker is an ex-
smoker the moment he puts down his last cigarette, and stays one until
he lights up again; a drinker becomes a teetotaler merely by abstain-
ing from one moment to the next. An overweight person, on the other
hand, has to make that same kind of heroic choice, then wait however
long it takes to lose all the excess weight before claiming success.

Therefore—unless you are a *very* slow reader—you have probably
not reached your ideal weight in the time between beginning to read
this book and coming to the end of it. You haven't yet started experiencing in your own life all the joys of being as thin as you want to be,
of glorying in your body rather than agonizing over its flaws. For most
dieters the train to the Promised Land stops here. Most diet books
think so, too; like fairy tales, they leave off at the point agreed upon
by convention: "Then she got thin and lived happily ever after."

The convention is so universal because up to this point everyone,
writers and readers alike, can agree upon what the goal is: lose weight.
After the weight is lost, confusion sets in. Are there further goals? If
so, what are they? It's easier to stop at a point at which the ground
seems firm beneath one's feet. This book won't stop there, however,
because beyond that point lie the most interesting issues and ideas of
all. The eternal quest for Getting Thin is fundamentally a question of
personal growth—that is, what kind of thin bodymind will you have?
What have you been practicing (experiencing over and over, getting
better and better at) as you lost your weight?

One of the things to notice about being overweight, being weight-conscious, being constantly on a diet, and so forth is how intensely self-involved one becomes. The "Big Book" of Alcoholics Anonymous characterizes the compulsive personality as "an extreme example of self-will run riot," and comments, "Any life run on self-will can hardly be a success." Our culture, however, explicitly condones bodily narcissism; diet books and articles magnify the reader's anxious self-concern for thousands and thousands of pages a year.

One article warned the dieter that he or she would receive the most compliments while losing; after the weight was gone friends and family would start taking the new body for granted, and soon stop paying extravagant compliments. You may gain your weight right back, the article admonished the reader, if you expect to be complimented constantly. I agree. Remember that being thin is normal—in other words, unremarkable—in a thin world. The question really is, Are you a person who would expect to have the world compliment you extravagantly for the rest of your life? In *Eating Disorders* Hilde Bruch discusses such people, whom she calls "thin fat people":

Such people, though they no longer look obese, are far from cured; they still resemble fat people with all their unsolved problems, conflicts, and exaggerated expectations. Only they no longer *show* their fat. [I call them] *Thin Fat People.* . . . Many women make a fetish of being thin and follow reducing diets without awareness or regard for the fact that they can do so only at the price of continuous strain and tension and some degree of ill health.

When we are obsessed with ourselves and our imperfections, there is just no time left over to pay much attention to anyone else, let alone to offer sympathetic help to someone who may desperately need it. The final step of the twelve-step "Anonymous" program of recovery is "Having had a spiritual awakening as the result of these steps, we tried to carry this message to [others] and to practice these principles in all our affairs." This is often expressed colloquially as "You can't keep it unless you give it away." In other words, you acquire the serenity necessary to conquer your own addictive behavior only by learning to be less self-centered. To "keep it" you need to practice, to continue spending time in self-subduing pursuits such as showing others, by personal example and counseling, how to solve their problems. "Anonymous" group members have learned to identify with, not vilify, others who suffer from their condition. Each of these programs envisions a truly "anonymous" (that is, ego-free) existence for its members, a self-disciplining goal that requires daily renewal.

When a person who was formerly what Dr. Rubin calls the Family Fat Center of Attention reduces to normal weight, the entire set of his or her family relationships is bound to change for the better. Since each of our lives is a dense matrix of relationships, it is axiomatic that when one member of a given network improves in body and mind the reverberations will be felt through everyone's lives like ripples in a pond. This has been true for our family, at least; I was always the family's element of disorder—habitually depressed, cranky, and self-pitying. Only when my mental health improved as my diet improved could I contribute anything meaningful to my family rather than diminish everyone else's happiness.

In due time we will be able to see that all bodies on earth fit into the general subject of "ecology"; that bodies are simply systems within systems. It will become clearer to us that there is a pattern and a structure to the world that does not have one's self at its center. No, wait; the pattern *does* have the self as epicenter, but in a way entirely different from egocentrism. Humanity as a whole can make significant progress only through alterations of individual consciousness, the effects of which then spread throughout each person's network of relationships. In truth, we are each other's environment; a balanced ecology is the health of the whole system. Stress is always spoken of as a nationwide problem, but it can be solved only at the individual level.

Our society is nothing more than the sum of our individual selves. Though our economic and political systems have frequently been criticized for their shortcomings, the inescapable truth about a marketplace economy and a participatory democracy is that they unerringly reflect our collective consciousness. The good news is that we get exactly what we demand; the bad news is that we are forced to live with the consequences of the insane choices we have been making so far. If we want the whole to improve, we must be ready to start at home, with ourselves. For overeaters this fact is undeniable. Fat parents would hate to have their children grow up to be obese, but their own bad eating habits create the demand that keeps the food-processing industry constantly manufacturing nonnourishing foodlike products (which one writer called "decoy food"). It was hypocritical of me, a fatty hooked on trash food, to lecture my children on good eating and to try to keep them away from sweets. My maternal instincts were sound, of course; I did not and do not want their lives blighted by a sugar addiction like mine. But as long as I was still *buying* the trash, secretly, to feed my hidden vice, I was guaranteeing that such products would never disappear. If you're still hooked on your favorite brand of candy bar or cupcake, then *you* are the reason it's there.

A culture is a set of agreements about how to do things, ritual actions and beliefs that constitute the "right" way to do and think (as "dieting" is a universally accepted preoccupation in our culture, at all social levels). A culture also agrees upon which of its members are to be considered heroes and which pariahs. Ours has overwhelmingly agreed to censure fat people; in fact, the consensus is such that even fat people themselves accept it. Overweight people tend to feel distaste for each other. People who were once fat but who have become thin almost always find themselves feeling superior to people who are still fat; everyone wants to play the "better than" game at every available opportunity. Every time I lost a few pounds, without fail I would look askance at my friends who were the same size as I had been; I only stopped the game when I'd gained the weight back and was not eligible to play any more. Sometimes it seemed to me that I operated in only two modes: binging out of control or holier-than-thou.

Only when fat people can see themselves as an "oppressed minority group" like other such groups will they be able to follow the others' example, realizing that the only possible first step is to jettison the paralyzing self-hatred that keeps the oppressed agreeing with the derogatory views of the oppressors. Being able to view overeating without judgment, as simply the organism's conditioned response to stress, is crucial. Surely we ought to be curious enough about ourselves and our motives to ask why our society continues to narrow its definition of bodily acceptability on several different fronts: weight, age, chic, and so forth. What is the point of paying attention only to youthful perfection if the truth is that we all get old?

Obviously, the people at the forefront in any attempt to change the culture's set of agreements will be, or at least should be, those who find themselves the victims of the present agreements. In a perverse sense we fat people should be profoundly grateful to our culture for sending us such a loud, clear, and unambiguous message: Being Fat is Wrong. Why is this an advantage? Well, it gets you closer to that personal cracking point where you're ready to give up in despair and accept a genuine solution. Think of the millions of problem drinkers in this country who will never be able to admit that they are alcoholics because our society permits them to think their addiction is only "being sophisticated" or "having fun"—an illusion fat people would never be permitted to sustain.

In fact, we who have spent time as compulsive overeaters have something uniquely valuable to contribute to our society and its mental health. Thin people may be astonished to hear that fat people have a lot to teach them, but they do. A great deal of human suffering originates in neurotic fears or hurts or shame that a person is simply too proud to acknowledge and must therefore bear alone. Fat people are those who have *had* to acknowledge their problems, at least on some level, for the simple reason that they were too visible to hide.

The corollary, however, is that we be able to identify with, not vilify, alcoholics and drug addicts and other compulsive members of our society. This may be difficult; we overeaters are noted for being law-abiding citizens, by virtue of the fact that our poison has not been judged an illegal substance. It may be almost impossible for a plump upper-middle-class matron to identify with the winos and junkies of Skid Row. But, like it or not, except for the arbitrary choice of poisonous substance all addicts are brothers and sisters under the skin. When you identify with the other compulsive people our society produces, you are led inevitably to one conclusion: if the method that cured you was improving the health of your body, increasing your self-esteem, learning to elicit beneficial feedback from your life circumstances, and keeping that sense of joy with yourself, then that is what everyone else needs, too. An extract from E. M. Forster's *A Passage to India* sums it up as well as any words could:

"Mr. Fielding, no one can ever realize how much kindness we Indians need, we do not even realize it ourselves. But we know when it has been given. We do not forget, though we may seem to. Kindness, more kindness, and even after that more kindness. I assure you it is the only hope."

Most of our apparent social and economic problems stem from one major source: cleaning up the waste and debris that a society accumulates when it doesn't pay enough attention to how people are feeling. As George Leonard observed, "Unaware of our own feelings, we can ignore the feelings of others, the urgent needs of the planet itself. The weaker we become, the more dangerous." The drug and alcoholism rehabilitation programs, welfare programs, job programs, and so forth are needed primarily because we don't care enough about each other not to let each other break down and need rehabilitation.

I once happened across the sentence "Despite our willingness to find technological remedies, the sense of failure survives." Why? Because we have not set the right priorities—human needs first—and therefore have willfully created a society that is not sufficiently nourishing to its members, whatever their social status. We have some strengths, true. No one has surpassed us in quantity and quality of material production. We have envisioned, then brought into being on the widest possible scale, a wondrous cornucopia of goods. But we still hunger for what has not been provided: a sense of purpose and emotional satisfaction. We had goals, and we reached them—but found them empty of meaning when we arrived. In a very basic sense, our society is a paradoxical mixture of gluttony and starvation.

We hear a lot about choices—that we are the luckiest people on earth because we have so many choices (read, a dizzying variety of consumer goods). It is a rather bizarre idea. None of our choices is free; each one of them carries its price. We just aren't aware enough even to know what the price is. We've set up our lives so that we think we are making choices when all we're really doing is being allowed to make *bad* choices. As an acquaintance of mine recently said, "The law of the survival of the fittest is still operating, and everyone who eats junk food just makes it work a little faster." In other words, those who are going to be doing the surviving around here are the people who don't make that particular choice.

Can a cheetah on the plains of Africa choose if he's going to run far enough every day to catch something to eat? No, he has the choice only if he's willing to starve. That choice is an absurdity, so of course he doesn't choose it. As a result of the running his body stays physically fit; a creature without minimal fitness won't be able to catch his prey and will soon be eliminated. For us, the invention of the automobile has given us the illusion that we have the choice of whether or not to move our bodies, and our endless inventiveness has created an array of new mini-choices to avoid movement. But the truth is that we have no more choice than does the cheetah; we have merely tricked out the choice leading to death so attractively that some of us are naive enough to deliberately opt for it. A perversion of the natural order, perhaps, but perhaps not. In our civilization it may be all for the best that the only ones to survive will be those that had the extraordinary intelligence to make the right choices even when the wrong ones were so available and alluring. Our present-day choices should not be seen as ends in themselves, but as interim contributions to our evolutionary potential. We make choices constantly; each one of them has meaning, and taken together they constitute the collective wisdom (or ignorance) of our society. That wisdom, measured against natural laws, is the sum total of our evolutionary capacity.

We simply must become wise enough to see that our present cultural agreements have become lethal not merely for an unlucky few, but for the majority of the population. Kenneth Pelletier quotes René Dubos, the wise writer on health and life, as observing: "Each civilization has its own kind of pestilence and can control it only by reforming itself." Ironically, our particular pestilence results from all too successfully achieving the goals we thought we wanted.

Gregory Bateson once commented that the evolutionary unit is not the organism alone, but the organism-in-its-environment. Knowing this, we are all the more duty bound to see the whole, without which "all the rest is desolation." At the moment we are like stunted houseplants—desert succulents growing in a gloomy den or tropical ferns in an arid living room. Under such conditions the creature doesn't die—it may survive for years—but it droops. One would never use it as an example of what was normal for that species. Our problem is that we have let our choices deform us to the extent that we no longer remember what "normal" looks or feels like, and we have thus become increasingly unable to diagnose our condition.

The fundamental issue is nutritional. Without remedies for our present nutritional deficiencies, all of the mutual kindness in the world won't be enough to save us. In fact, as earlier chapters have argued, kindness (as well as mental health) *is* a nutritional issue. I spoke earlier of the victims of a given culture's agreements being those who should be most inclined to work for change; when we add nutritional factors to social ones, the list of victims becomes almost as large as the total population.

In *Food Pollution* Gene Marine and Judith Van Allen put the case very directly: "Things are not all right just because we are told, over and over again, that they are. The feeling at first opens a great void before us . . . but that feeling, once the initial shock is over, is maturity, for an individual or for the human race. . . . We cannot—in fact we must not—take it for granted that *anything* on the grocery shelf is healthy, FDA approval or not." Much of that book discusses the carcinogenicity of food additives and coloring agents and the toxicity of pesticides, but it also rails against the food processors' constant tampering with natural ingredients to make "food products," an insanity when seen from an ecological perspective: "[Eating] is an ecological process, with each part bearing on each other part in ways that are understood today in only the dimmest of fashions. It has evolved as a part of our own incredibly complex inner-ecological evolution. We tamper with it at our peril." Leonard, Hofer, and Pritikin's evaluation of the majority of today's food products in *Live Longer Now* echoes Marine and Van Allen's: "When food has been changed so that it no longer nourishes your body or becomes dangerous to your health, we call it garbage. . . . By our definition, much of what is being sold as food on your supermarket's shelves is not really food at all. It is garbage. It is garbage handsomely packaged and labeled as food, but it is garbage all the same."

Once I was asked to speak at a meeting of the Los Angeles chapter of the American Chemical Society. At dinner beforehand my husband and I began chatting with a man who identified himself as a "food chemist" in charge of developing various "food products" to be manufactured by one of the large food-processing companies. When we asked him what was the first step in that process, he told us that it was to decide what the "food" should look like. After the appearance of the food and the design of the container had been worked out, the product was test-marketed to see if there would be sufficient demand to make it worthwhile to produce. My husband and I were utterly dumbfounded; we thought we were fairly cynical about the food-processing industry, but even we weren't prepared for such a bald statement about the process. In fact, we later read a newspaper article about an even less nutritionally oriented motive than those the chemist had mentioned for the development of new food products: *gaining more shelf space!* Apparently, what the food companies care about most is how much of the total display space on a grocer's shelves will be devoted to their products; more products take up more room and thus dominate the display.

The advertising of "decoy food" is highly sophisticated propaganda. Because much of our economy is based on advertising, and we are so saturated with it, we have simply come to expect exaggerated claims and minor falsehoods to be part of every broadcasted message we hear. But, as I said earlier, the only perspective that matters is evolutionary: are the choices we're making helping us or hindering us in our wish to survive? When a well-known actress tells us in a television commercial that Hostess fruit pies, Twinkies, and Ding Dongs are wholesome, it's a seductive message spoken by an attractive woman, but from an evolutionary perspective it's nonsense—another blandishment we *must* be intelligent enough to dismiss, or risk the survival of our species.

But the very effectiveness of our relentless, multibillion-dollar advertising raises some basic questions about the morality of the persuasion methods used to reach (or exploit, if you wish) our least discriminating and most vulnerable consumers: children. As food products proliferate, they invariably crowd the more nourishing, but less profitable, food commodities off the shelves. Marine and Van Allen warn parents not to feed their children popular breakfast cereals, pointing out that they exist not because of their nutritional value. "They are manufactured solely because they are by far the most profitable 'foods' produced in America." They also report the results of a very disturbing study:

Dr. Philip Jeans of Iowa State University's College of Medicine did some looking around, and discovered that in our "well-fed" society, a great many children have average weight for their height and age, but they lack good muscles and good posture. . . . The kids get plenty of calories. But not enough of them come from animal-protein foods nor from high-protein vegetables. . . . Muscles don't achieve what Dr. Jeans called "the expected normal growth"— and you'll notice that he didn't say the *optimal* growth.

After making a superhuman effort to obtain pure foods, many parents of hyperactive children are finding out for themselves, despite all the claims of the food industry, that their children are much healthier and easier to manage on a diet free of additives. The tragedy is that they should have to work so hard and unremittingly to obtain for their children what should be every child's natural right.

It seems unimaginable now, but there was a time a decade or so ago when we "didn't know" about pollution. We still thought it was possible to "throw things away." We thought that free enterprise permitted the manufacturers of industrial chemicals to produce their products in unlimited amounts and disperse them widely in the environment. Thankfully, we're not so naive in this area any more; we understand that the moral issue of our common survival must override the individual's right to make a profit by harming others.

We may be on the verge of a similar awakening with respect to nutritional issues. We may become aware of the absurdity of entrusting the delivery of our food—the only raw material we have for constructing our bodies—to food-processing companies that want to profit by altering the food into "food products," substituting cheaper and shoddier ingredients whenever possible. It is not a sane system, and its result is not sane minds in healthy bodies. Even a small change in our present habits ought to make a big difference in how people feel and act, which could have a synergistic effect. The practical application to modern society of what we know about nutrition, as Dr. Frank G. Boudreau says in Brennan and Mulligan's *Nutrigenetics,* could produce "an enormous improvement in public health, at least equal to that which resulted when the germ theory of infectious disease was made the basis of public health and medical work." But if we are going to reap these rewards, we must be willing to demand what we need. As Jim Hightower pointed out in *Eat Your Heart Out: How Food Profiteers Victimize the Consumer,* "There is a point at which people must say 'No more.' Big-business technologies and systems will push you around to fit their needs until you finally refuse to be pushed. . . . At the very least, you have to be a human being, willing to ask 'Why?' whenever big business and government demand that you adjust to their version of progress, and willing to say 'No!' if the answer does not satisfy you."

Working on the problem of making our society more humane is the exact counterpart to the subject of most of this book, working on the problem of making a body thinner. Both a person and a society are cybernetic systems, and identical factors operate in each. The first issue is mental tools; new ones may be needed to become aware of both the dimensions of the problem and the paths toward a solution. As Joseph Chilton Pearce observed, "The way out is a way *beyond*, not a rehashing of ruined ingredients."

The second issue is the importance of seeing the whole. Like the body, the society is a complex whole maintaining itself in equilibrium. The equilibrium may not be particularly healthy, but it's a *given:* the sum of a long series of prior choices. Being unable to see the whole produces all kinds of difficulties. First is self-centeredness, as exemplified by our society's endemic "me-first" attitude, which is self-will run riot on a giant scale. For as long as we can remember, our society has turned all its energies toward What I Want at the expense of What I Need, and it is now being forced to confront the results. The second difficulty is a belief in the efficacy of easy solutions—treating symptoms instead of diseases. This is just as tempting on the social as on the individual level: tinker a bit here, spend some money there, start another government program. All are dead ends. The third difficulty of partial sight may be harder to comprehend: it is the tendency to see the *system's* difficulties as single problems unrelated to one another. Thus, for example, it is possible to see alcoholics, drug addicts, child beaters, and criminals as "problems" without understanding the inescapable connection of these problems with stress in the nutritional and emotional environment. It doesn't occur to us that there could be any connection between the wino or the junkie and the president of a big national cookie company. Conversely, it is wrong to think of the giant food-processing companies as the "villains" or the "problem" without understanding that they could not possibly exist if we had not collectively willed them into being.

When we understand that only seeing whole will do, we begin to be ready to discard some of our cultural blind spots. We are less likely to condemn certain discrete parts of the system's problem on spurious grounds; we are less comfortable with partial fix-it solutions. Having seen that the primary issue is information exchange within the system, we become slightly less dogmatic materialists; seeing the dynamic, self-correcting quality of the system's equilibrium, we better understand the notion of process.

It's necessary to keep in mind Bateson's definition of the "interlocking circuits of contingency" on which all life depends. Everything is connected to everything else. Just as awareness helped us learn more about formerly invisible aspects of ourselves, so it can help make manifest the innumerable circuits of contingency the system comprises.

After we've become aware of the equilibrium of the system we have, and see that we've made it what it is now, we can then ask how it might change for the better. The central issue, as always, is cybernetic: what are we paying attention to—in other words, what authorities do we follow and why do we listen to them? Right now we've surrendered much too much authority to three groups whose vested interests do not coincide with our best bodily health: doctors, the food-processing companies, and the advertising industry. The system is unhealthy as it stands now, and it will not improve until each of us understands that we have the right to demand something better.

As I waited in a doctor's outer office one day, I happened to pick up a glossy, expensive-looking magazine entitled *Diversion: For Physicians at Leisure.* The editorial content touted on the cover ranged from a wine-drinking tour of New York state to a posh holiday in the Caribbean. Inside, the first page was a full-page ad extolling the automotive elegance of the Jaguar. Immediately following were several colorful double-page spreads, one for a "bowel-management program" using Fleet, a liquid laxative preparation, and another for Ritalin, a drug to combat depression in adults and hyperactivity in children. Interestingly enough, a simple, inexpensive program of eating natural unprocessed foods could do much toward solving both problems, though such a regime would sidestep entirely the economic structure in which a Jaguar is a well-earned reward.

But there is hope. Doctors are people, and the basis of each doctor's practice is his or her personal relationship with each patient. We can make our wants known in a highly personal way, without having to fight bureaucracy or red tape. We need only speak up. As Dr. Tom Ferguson, the editor of *Medical Self-Care: Access to Tools,* said in an interview, "If a doctor receives letters from 10 patients asking him to change the way he deals with them, he won't ignore it." One of the first things to ask for is a greater awareness of and sensitivity to nutritional issues.

When I started writing this book, I felt a certain sense of resentment that enormous food-processing companies and giant advertising firms should be using their considerable economic power to seduce people into eating food that was not good for them. Then, however, I realized that this was not the issue at all. Advertising has the power to reach only those who have not yet decided they are no longer interested in this particular seduction. Cigarette smoking is a good case in point. Many smokers, even formerly heavy smokers, have stopped smoking because they are convinced it is dangerous. Their decision is final. Tobacco companies could increase their advertising budgets a hundredfold without being able to reach these people, who have decided they want to be healthy instead. Many people have already made the same kind of decision with respect to the food they want to eat. One magazine article I read commented that the spreading interest in athletic competition in this country was forcing the issue of healthy eating for many people, far in advance of current medical or food industry thinking or recommendations.

The statement that every one of our nationwide problems is something that can be solved only at the individual level is not pessimistic; on the contrary, the fact that the issue is one of *individual* consciousness is a cause for great optimism, since changes in consciousness can occur virtually instantaneously when the proper information is made available. George Leonard says it as well as anyone could: "Behind each improvement that can be attributed to 'technology,' there lies a powerful human intentionality, the purpose of which is evolution, transcendence, transformation. . . . Ultimately, human intentionality is the most powerful evolutionary force on this planet."

Each of our individual decisions, then, contributes to the evolutionary potential of the whole. We may tend to feel slightly apprehensive; how can we know if our decisions are leading toward evolutionary fitness or not? The only sure criterion is whether the choice leads to peace of mind and body. If so, it's on the right track.

We are so accustomed to our materialist paradigm that we have difficulty with any explanation of reality that seems "spiritual" in nature; we seem to prefer *spiritual* to mean "in heaven" with "God." It seems clear, however, that the cybernetics issues with which this book deals—the questions of transmission and feedback of information— are as close to a secular concept of spirituality as we need to come. First read Gregory Bateson (in Brand's *Two Cybernetic Frontiers*) on the question of evolutionary adaptation: "Natural selection does not deal with you, who obviously don't last very long, it deals with biological ideas in genomes—programs. The unit of evolution is ideas, it's not organisms." Then read a mystically minded writer on the same subject: "All the good food in the world is not enough to make even a single person truly healthy and happy. Health and the sense of well-being which accompanies it is the result of attuning oneself to natural laws and living by the principles those laws make clear. This harmonizing of one's life is spiritual in nature" (quoted in McClure and Lane's *Cooking for Consciousness*).

Our quest for an evolutionarily sane life lived in harmony with natural laws can result in spiritual goals, though these would have to be defined as bodily experiences, since as mere grand-sounding concepts they have no operational reality. The possibilities include the following: to replace our pervasive anxiety with an ongoing serenity; to be able to relax and "let go"; to replace boredom with absorbed attention to whatever we are doing; to replace self-obsession with caring for others and a sense of community. They will do for a start.

References

Abrahamson, E. M., and Pezet, A. W. *Body, Mind, and Sugar*. New York: Pyramid, 1971.

Adams, Ruth, and Murray, Frank. *Megavitamin Therapy*. New York: Larchmont Books, 1973.

Airola, Paavo. *Hypoglycemia: A Better Approach*. Phoenix, Ariz.: Health Plus Publishers, 1977.

Alcoholics Anonymous (the "Big Book"). 3rd ed. New York: Alcoholics Anonymous World Services, 1976.

Alexander, F. Matthias. *The Resurrection of the Body: The Writings of F. Matthias Alexander*. Selected and introduced by Edward Maisel. New York: University Books, 1969.

Alexander, Franz. *Psychosomatic Medicine*. New York: W. W. Norton, 1950.

Ashby, W. Ross. *Design for a Brain*. 2nd ed. London: Chapman & Hall, 1960.

Atkins, Robert C. *Dr. Atkins' Diet Revolution*. New York: David McKay, 1972.

Atkins, Robert C., and Linde, Shirley. *Dr. Atkins' Superenergy Diet*. New York: Bantam, 1978.

Bach, Richard. *A Gift of Wings*. New York: Dell, 1974.

Bach, Richard. *Jonathan Livingston Seagull*. New York: Macmillan, 1970.

Barlow, Wilfred. *The Alexander Technique*. New York: Knopf, 1976.

Bateson, Gregory. *Mind and Nature: A Necessary Unity*. New York: E. P. Dutton, 1979.

Bateson, Gregory. *Steps to an Ecology of Mind*. New York: Ballantine, 1972.

Beller, Anne Scott. *Fat and Thin: A Natural History of Obesity*. New York: Farrar, Straus and Giroux, 1977.

Bennett, Hal, and Samuels, Mike. *Be Well*. New York: Random House, 1975.

Bertherat, Thérèse, and Bernstein, Carol. *The Body Has Its Reasons*. New York: Pantheon, 1977.

Bonow, Raysa Rose. *How to Be a Thin Person*. New York: Random House, 1977.

Brand, Stewart. *Two Cybernetic Frontiers*. New York: Random House, 1974.

Brennan, R. O., and Mulligan, William C. *Nutrigenetics*. New York: Evans, 1975.

Brown, Barbara. *New Mind, New Body*. New York: Bantam, 1975.

Brown, Barbara. *Stress and the Art of Biofeedback*. New York: Bantam, 1978.

Brown, Barbara. Interviewed in Nathaniel Lande, *Mindstyles, Lifestyles*.

Bruch, Hilde. *Eating Disorders*. New York: Basic Books, 1973.

Castaneda, Carlos. *Journey to Ixtlan*. New York: Pocket Books, 1974.

Castaneda, Carlos. *The Second Ring of Power*. New York: Simon & Schuster, 1977.

Castaneda, Carlos. *A Separate Reality*. New York: Pocket Books, 1972.

Castaneda, Carlos. *Tales of Power*. New York: Pocket Books, 1976.

Cheraskin, E.; Ringsdorf, W. M.; and Clark, J. W. *Diet and Disease*. Emmaus, Penn.: Rodale Books, 1968.

Christians, George F. *The Compulsive Overeater*. Garden City, N. Y.: Doubleday, 1978.

Cormillot, Alberto. *Thin Forever*. New York: Henry Regnery, 1976.

Corriere, Richard, and Hart, Joseph. *The Dream Makers*. New York: Bantam, 1978.

Daniels, Victor, and Horowitz, Laurence J. *Being and Caring*. San Francisco: San Francisco Book Co., 1976.

Dass, Ram. Interviewed by Calvin Fentress in *New Times*, September 4, 1978.

Davis, Adelle. *Let's Eat Right to Keep Fit*. New York: New American Library, 1970.

Deikman, Arthur J. "The Meaning of Everything." In *The Nature of Human Consciousness*, edited by Robert E. Ornstein. New York: Viking, 1973.

Deutsch, Ronald M. *Realities of Nutrition*. Palo Alto, Calif.: Bull Publishing Co., 1976.

Diane Arbus. An Aperture Monograph. New York: Museum of Modern Art, 1972.

Didion, Joan. "On Self-Respect." In *Slouching Towards Bethlehem*. New York: Dell, 1968.

Dijkstra, Edsger. Interviewed by Michael W. Cashman in *Datamation*, May 1977.

Dillard, Annie. *Pilgrim at Tinker Creek*. New York: Harper's Magazine Press, 1974.

Dufty, William. *Sugar Blues*. New York: Warner, 1975.

Dychtwald, Ken. *Body-mind*. New York: Jove Publications, 1977.

Dyer, Wayne. "Stress! New Ways to Handle It." *Family Circle*, November 20, 1978.

Dyer, Wayne. *Your Erroneous Zones*. New York: Funk & Wagnalls, 1976.

Ellerbroek, W. C. "Language, Thought, and Disease." *The Coevolution Quarterly*, Spring 1978.

Ferguson, Tom. Interviewed in the *Los Angeles Times*, Section IV, February 28, 1979.

Frederick, Carl. *est: Playing the Game the New Way*. New York: Dell, 1974.

Friedman, Meyer, and Rosenman, Ray H. *Type A Behavior and Your Heart*. New York: Knopf, 1974.

Gallwey, Timothy. *Inner Tennis*. New York: Random House, 1976.

Gallwey, Timothy. Interviewed by Tony Schwartz in *New Times*, November 26, 1976.

Gatty, Ronald. *The Body Clock Diet*. New York: Simon & Schuster, 1978.

Gladwin, Thomas. *East Is a Big Bird: Navigation and Logic on Puluwat Atoll.* Cambridge, Mass.: Harvard University Press, 1970.

Gerrard, Don. *One Bowl.* New York: Random House, 1974.

Glasser, William. *Positive Addiction.* New York: Harper & Row, 1976.

Golas, Thaddeus. *The Lazy Man's Guide to Enlightenment.* Palo Alto, Calif.: The Seed Center, 1972.

Gombrich, E. H. *The Sense of Order: A Study in the Psychology of Decorative Art.* Ithaca, N.Y.: Cornell University Press, 1979.

Gould, Roger. Interviewed in the *Los Angeles Times,* Section IV, July 5, 1978.

Gross, Amy. "Fat Control." *Mademoiselle,* August 1973.

Gross, Amy. "The New Discipline." *Vogue,* January 1979.

Gwinup, Grant. *Energetics.* New York: Bantam, 1970.

Hassett, Marilyn. Interviewed in *Mademoiselle,* January 1979.

Hawken, Paul. *The Magic of Findhorn.* New York: Bantam, 1976.

Heisel, Dorelle. *The Biofeedback Exercise Book.* New York: New American Library, 1974.

Hightower, Jim. *Eat Your Heart Out.* New York: Crown, 1975.

Hittleman, Richard. *Guide to Yoga Meditation.* New York: Bantam, 1969.

Ichazo, Oscar. *Arica Psychocalisthenics.* New York: Simon & Schuster, 1976.

Jansen, John, and Catlett, Joyce. *The Love Diet Strategy.* Los Angeles: Glendon House, 1978.

Jordan, Henry A.; Levitz, Leonard S.; and Kimbrell, Gordon M. *Eating Is Okay!* New York: New American Library, 1976.

Keleman, Stanley. *Your Body Speaks Its Mind.* New York: Pocket Books, 1976.

Laing, R. D. *The Divided Self.* New York: Pantheon, 1969.

Lamb, Lawrence E. *Metabolics.* New York: Harper & Row, 1974.

Lande, Nathaniel. *Mindstyles, Lifestyles.* Los Angeles: Price/Stern/Sloan, 1976.

Leonard, George. *The Ultimate Athlete.* New York: Avon, 1977.

Leonard, Jon N.; Hofer, J. L.; and Pritikin, N. *Live Longer Now.* New York: Charter Books, 1974.

LeShan, Eda. *Winning the Losing Battle.* New York: Crowell, 1979.

Liebman, Joshua Loth. *Peace of Mind.* New York: Simon & Schuster, 1946.

Lindner, Peter. *Mind over Platter.* Los Angeles: Wilshire Book Company, 1975.

Lowen, Alexander. *The Betrayal of the Body.* New York: Collier, 1967.

Maezumi, Hakuyu Taizan. *The Way of Everyday Life.* Los Angeles: Center Publications, 1979.

Maltz, Maxwell. *Psycho-cybernetics.* New York: Pocket Books, 1976.

Mandell, Arnold. Interviewed by Jonathan Black in *The Runner,* April 1979.

Marine, Gene, and Van Allen, Judith. *Food Pollution.* New York: Holt, Rinehart and Winston, 1972.

Masters, George, and Browning, Norma Lee. *The Masters Way to Beauty.* New York: New American Library, 1977.

Mayer, Jean. *Overweight: Causes, Cost, and Control.* Englewood Cliffs, N.J.: Prentice-Hall, 1968.

McClure, Joy, and Layne, Kendall. *Cooking for Consciousness.* Denver: Ananda Marga Publications, 1976.

Miller, Don. *Bodymind: The Whole Person Health Book.* Englewood Cliffs, N.J.: Prentice-Hall, 1974.

Murphy, Michael. *Golf in the Kingdom.* New York: Dell, 1972.

Newbold, H. L. *Dr. Newbold's Revolutionary New Discoveries About Weight Loss.* New York: Rawson Associates, 1977.

Newman, Mildred, and Berkowitz, Bernard. *How to Be Your Own Best Friend.* New York: Random House, 1971.

Null, Gary, and Null, Steve. *Alcohol and Nutrition.* New York: Pyramid, 1977.

Ohsawa, George. *Macrobiotics: An Invitation to Health and Happiness.* Oroville, Calif.: George Ohsawa Macrobiotic Foundation, 1971.

Palm, J. Daniel. *Diet Away Your Stress, Tension, and Anxiety.* New York: Pocket Books, 1977.

Page, Melvin E., and Abrams, H. Leon. *Your Body Is Your Best Doctor.* New Canaan, Conn.: Keats Publishing, 1976.

Pearce, Joseph Chilton. *The Crack in the Cosmic Egg.* New York: Pocket Books, 1973.

Peele, Stanton, and Brodsky, Archie. *Love and Addiction.* New York: New American Library, 1975.

Pelletier, Kenneth R. *Mind as Healer, Mind as Slayer.* New York: Dell, 1977.

Pritikin, Nathan. Interviewed in *Family Circle,* November 20, 1978.

Pritikin, Nathan. Interviewed in *The New York Times Book Review,* July 1, 1979.

Progoff, Ira. *At a Journal Workshop.* New York: Dialogue House Library, 1975.

Progoff, Ira. Interviewed by Jack Fincher in *Human Behavior,* November 1975.

Reich, Laurence. *From Fat to Skinny.* New York: Wyden Books, 1977.

Rohé, Fred. *The Zen of Running.* New York: Random House, 1974.

de Ropp, Robert. *The Master Game.* New York: Dell, 1968.

Rubin, Theodore Isaac. *Compassion and Self-Hate: An Alternative to Despair.* New York: David McKay, 1975.

Rubin, Theodore Isaac. *Forever Thin.* New York: Gramercy, 1970.

Scarf, Maggie. *Body, Mind, Behavior.* New York: Dell, 1977.

Schauf, George E. *Think Thin.* New York: Fawcett, 1970.

Schiff, Martin M. *Dr. Schiff's Miracle Weight-Loss Guide.* West Nyack, N.Y.: Parker, 1974.

Schoenstadt, David A. *The San Francisco Weight-Loss Method.* New York: Arthur Fields, 1975.

Schutz, Will. *Profound Simplicity*. New York: Bantam, 1979.

Seligson, Marcia, and *Cosmopolitan*. *Cosmopolitan's Super Diets & Exercise Guide*. New York: Cosmopolitan Books, 1973.

Selye, Hans. *The Stress of Life*. New York: McGraw-Hill, 1956.

Selye, Hans. *Stress without Distress*. New York: New American Library, 1975.

Selye, Hans. Preface to Nathaniel Lande, *Mindstyles, Lifestyles*.

Silva, José. *The Silva Mind Control Method*. New York: Pocket Books, 1978.

Smith, Adam. *Powers of Mind*. New York: Random House, 1975.

Solomon, Neil, and Sheppard, Sally. *The Truth about Weight Control*. New York: Stein and Day, 1971.

Spiegel, Herbert. Interviewed by David Black in *New Times,* April 29, 1977.

Suinn, Richard. Interviewed by Amy Gross in *Mademoiselle,* May 1977.

Suzuki, Shunryu. *Zen Mind, Beginner's Mind*. New York and Tokyo: John Weatherhill, 1970.

Tennov, Dorothy. *Super Self: A Woman's Guide to Self-Management*. New York: Harcourt Brace Jovanovich, 1977.

Thomas, Lewis. *The Medusa and the Snail*. New York: Viking, 1979.

Trungpa, Chögyma. *Cutting through Spiritual Materialism*. Boulder, Colo.: Shambhala Publications, 1973.

Twelve Steps and Twelve Traditions. New York: Alcoholics Anonymous World Services, 1952.

Tyler, H. Richard, and Dawson, David M., eds. *Current Neurology*. Boston: Houghton Mifflin, 1979.

Tyson, Richard, and Walker, Jay R. *The Meditation Diet*. Chicago: Playboy Press, 1976.

Watson, George. *Nutrition and Your Mind*. New York: Harper & Row, 1972.

Weinberg, George. *The Action Approach: How Your Personality Developed and How You Can Change It*. New York: World, 1969.

Weinberg, George. *Self-Creation*. New York: St. Martin's, 1978.

Westin, Jeanne Eddy. *The Thin Book*. Newport Beach, Calif.: CompCare Publications, 1978.

White, E. B. *The Essays of E. B. White*. New York: Harper & Row, 1977.

Wiener, Norbert. *Cybernetics*. 2nd ed. Cambridge, Mass.: The MIT Press, 1961.

Winter, J. A. *Why We Get Sick: The Origins of Illness and Anxiety*. New York: Weathervane Books, 1962.

Yudkin, John. *Sweet and Dangerous*. New York: Bantam, 1973.

Yudkin, John. *Lose Weight, Feel Great!* New York: Larchmont Books, 1974.

Other good books for weight-losers from CompCare Publications

Break Out of Your Fat Cell, *The Holistic Mind/Body Guide to Permanent Weight Loss,* Jeane Eddy Westin, author of the best selling *The Thin Book.* This looks at the problem of overweight from a "whole person" point of view, relating successful weight loss to a positive self-image and offering practical strategies for survival in a thin chauvinist society. It helps weight-losers live complete, satisfying lives while they take off the pounds. *Quality paperback.*

Compulsive Overeater, Bill B. An interpretation of the Twelve Steps of Alcoholics Anonymous (AA) especially for compulsive overeaters, this is an important book for those who are serious about losing their extra pounds — forever. Many thousands of overeaters have heard Bill B., who lives in California and lectures to standing room only audiences all over the country, share the way he works the Program and how he has maintained his seventy-five-pound weight loss for over ten years. Back to press four times in the first six months after publication! *Hardcover.*

A Day at a Time. This familiar, pocket-size CompCare classic, with its rust cover and gold title, now has a quarter of a million copies in print. These daily readings — thoughts, prayers, and memorable phrases for coping with life's complexities — are helpful for anyone, but especially for those working Twelve-Step Programs. Its wise words are passwords to serenity for the thousands who have made this little book a bedside or a carry-along source of strength. Jane Thomas Noland, author of *Laugh It Off,* wrote the "Today I Pray" and "Today I Will Remember" thoughts. For gifts, "abstinence" anniversaries, other special moments, choose the deluxe cover in padded burgundy leathergrained vinyl. *Hardcover.*

Laugh It Off, *A Self-discovery Workbook for Weight-losers,* Jane Thomas Noland. Used widely by individual weight-losers and weight-loss groups. Witty essays, cartoons, slogans, jingles and puns underline a valuable message — that shedding pounds is a positive experience. This pep-talks wishful shrinkers into losing the equivalent of half a twin-bed mattress or a truck tire. It offers *actual* ways (along with a *trick* way — flip-page animation) to make the scale go down! *Quality paperback.*

Mom, How Come I'm Not Thin? Bill and Enid Bluestein, illustrated by Susan Kennedy. Especially for ages 7 to 11. Winner of the Brandeis University Library Trust Award for Achievement in Children's Literature. Any overweight child who feels left behind in a thin world will find comfort in this gentle, sensitively illustrated story about 10-year-old Dolly. Pediatricians and counselors have welcomed this book. So have frustrated parents of chubby children, who find it's the long-needed answer to that question sometimes too painful to be asked out loud, "Mom, how come I'm not thin?" *Hardcover, picture book format.*

The Thin Book, *365 Daily Aids for Fat-free, Guilt-free, Binge-free Living,* Jeane Eddy Westin. Grateful weight-losers the world over have taken this book to heart and found daily inspiration in it, no matter what kind of weight-loss program they are following. This much-loved book, with over 85,000 in print, strikes at the core of the overweight's problem — sagging motivation — and keeps its readers on a thinning course. Excerpted by *Cosmopolitan* magazine in English- and foreign-language editions. *Quality paperback.*

This Will Drive You Sane, Bill L. Little, Foreword by Albert Ellis. A warm-hearted therapist with a towering sense of humor, known for his on-the-air counseling sessions over CBS Radio KMOX out of St. Louis, backhandedly shows how to get rid of problems by explaining, in droll detail, how to *produce* them. Misery is not simply a state of being, but an art to be developed — and wallowed in! This humorous approach to everyday problems can ease the stress that often leads to overweight. *Quality paperback.*

The Twelve Steps for Everyone . . . who really wants them. Originally written to interpret AA's Program for members of Emotional Health Anonymous (EHA), this sensitive book can help anyone find strength and healing through the Twelve Steps. Individuals as well as groups have found this interpretation of the Twelve Steps — with over 100,000 in print — easy to understand and apply. *Quality paperback.*

The Year Santa Got Thin, Enid and Bill Bluestein. A modern folktale in high-spirited rhyme, for all ages for all seasons, tells how Santa decides to change his shape and his image. This tall *thin* tale about pride and pudginess appeals at many levels as it smuggles in some good information about losing weight, vanity, and tampering with traditions. Brilliantly illustrated by Joe Pearson, it is a perfect gift for a family — yours or a friend's. *Hardcover, picture book format.*

All of the above books are published by and available from CompCare Publications. None is either endorsed or opposed by the author of this book. Ask us to send you a free CompCare Publications catalog of quality books and other materials emphasizing a positive approach to life's problems for young people and adults on a broad range of topics. If you have questions, call us toll free at 800/328-3330. (Minnesota residents: Call 612/559-4800.)

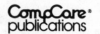

CompCare®
publications

2415 Annapolis Lane, Minneapolis, Minnesota 55441
a division of Comprehensive Care Corporation